Cliff Temple has been ... years, and qualified as ... since helped hundreds ... standards, as well as ... previous best-selling b... *Marathon*, *Jogging for Fitness and Pleasure*, *Running from A to Z.*

Among his most successful female athletes have been Shireen Bailey, who was an Olympic 1500 metres finalist for Britain in Seoul in 1988, and Sarah Rowell, a 1984 Olympic representative, World Student Games champion and former British record-holder for the marathon.

Temple, now 43, has been athletics correspondent of *The Sunday Times* since 1969, and has reported five Olympic Games for the newspaper. He is also coaching editor and columnist for *Running* magazine.

He and his wife Clare live in Hythe, East Kent, where she is chairman of Folkestone Athletic Club. They have three sons and one daughter.

# THE PERFECT END

## A Better Bottom in 10 Weeks

by

*Cliff Temple*

Queen Anne Press
Futura

A *Queen Anne Press*/Futura BOOK

First published in Great Britain in 1990 by
Queen Anne Press/Futura, a division of
Macdonald & Co (Publishers) Ltd
Orbit House
1 New Fetter Lane
London
EC4A 1AR

A member of Maxwell Macmillan Pergamon Publishing
Corporation

All photographs by Mark Shearman

Cover illustration by Richard Dunn

*Grateful thanks to Olympic finalist Shireen Bailey for
demonstrating the exercises and isocises for the photographic
section.*

ISBN 0 7088 4336 0

Typeset by Leaper & Gard Ltd, Bristol, England
Printed and bound in Great Britain by
BPCC Hazell Books
Aylesbury, Bucks, England
Member of BPCC Ltd

Dedicated to every female who has ever intended to start making her bottom trimmer tomorrow, with the humble suggestion that she could even start today . . .

# $-$INTRODUCTIO$N-$

$K$ate had already managed two laps of Tesco's before she succumbed. The mineral water and the fresh carrots, the low fat margarine and the Ryvita were already in her trolley, fairly low down. The other family necessities followed: the cereal with the free plastic toy, the chocolate spread and the beef and onion crisps.

But by the second circuit, when Stephen, five, and Terry, three and a half, had their third fight and brought the whole of the loo-roll special-offer display crashing down and rolling everywhere, the temptation proved too great. As she embarrassedly hustled them out, she dropped into the trolley, with a sprinkling of guilt and resignation, the box of walnut whips and the twin-pack of Mars bars which she had walked past so quickly 20 minutes earlier.

As a final afterthought while she queued at the check-out, she noticed on the counter a women's magazine with a cover photo of a trim, young lady (no children, no supermarket trolley). The cover proclaimed 'A New You in a Month with our Amazing New Diet!'. It struck the right chord at the right time. Kate picked it up and put it in the trolley, wedging it between the Mars bars and the diet Cokes. Only when she got it home did she remember she'd bought exactly the same magazine the previous week.

That dull rumbling sound as Sue made her way from Embankment Underground Station to Charing Cross could have been the 5.24 to Dartford moving out of platform 2. Or it could have been her stomach. It was now 21 hours and 17 minutes since she had last eaten anything substantial.

Catching sight of herself in the wardrobe mirror just before she went to bed the previous night she had (once again) vowed to lose weight. She had deliberately stayed in bed that morning, avoiding the temptation of breakfast, until the minimum possible time remained for her to get dressed, washed and walk the short distance to the station.

During the mid-morning coffee break in the City office where she worked she had made an excuse to pop out for a moment. At lunch-time she bought herself just one low-fat plain yoghurt, and left half of it. At tea time she asked for hers without milk, and left most of it. Now, 21 hours and 18 minutes since her last meal, she was beginning to feel slightly dizzy and faint. Her head ached. Her stomach rumbled again.

For a moment, she told herself that it had been a triumph of willpower, that she had got through a whole day at work consuming practically nothing. But then honesty prevailed: she knew she was not tackling the problem the right way. She knew that simply starving herself was not the best solution, nor the healthiest. And, above all, she felt so bloody hungry.

As she crossed the station concourse, the aroma of cheeseburgers and chips drifted across from the Casey Jones burger bar, reminding her of food gone by. There were two minutes before her train left. There was no one waiting at the confectionery kiosk, so she suddenly detoured on her way to the ticket barrier, fumbling for a pound coin in her purse. Moments later, clutching a Twix bar and a can of Coke, she hurried down the platform to find a place to stand on the train; the seats had all been taken ages ago.

As the train rattled and jerked across the points at London Bridge, Sue guiltily took a bite at the Twix bar.

She scarcely noticed her stomach cheering. Instead she was thinking: Surely there's a better way?

The Baroness was used to people looking at her, for she had that supreme confidence which comes with being born royal. Her hair was always immaculately groomed, her make-up subtle, yet expertly applied.

But as she glided up the escalator at Harrods, the smart black suit she wore could not disguise the problem she reluctantly, and perhaps unknowingly, shared with millions of others born in humbler circumstances. She assumed the long glances she was attracting from those around her were because of who she was. She was only partly right. The others were from women who had just been reassured in the best possible way that the pear-shaped problem was obviously not surmountable simply through the money and status they lacked.

Perhaps, after all, the solution really could be found purely through motivation and determination. And they cost nothing.

# – 1 –

Do you really want to spend the rest of your life trying to follow an apparently never-ending diet of lettuce leaves and bran flakes? Must you slavishly follow another 'incredible new diet' in order to shape an Incredible New You? Is it really necessary to spend so many hours every day with your stomach rumbling, ravenous with hunger, guiltily dreaming of a pink iced cream bun, in order to recapture the figure you may have inadvertently let slip?

Of course not. For the chief misconception generated by so many of those super-duper diet plans is that *only* by changing your nutritional intake to something akin to that of a constipated rabbit can you ever hope to become that slim, trim person you would like to see every morning in your bedroom mirror. That, of course, is nonsense.

There really is a better, healthier way of ensuring that the zips on your size 12 (or even size 10) dresses do up again, and that you can once more fasten the buttons on your favourite pair of tight Levi 501s without slicing yourself fore and aft.

Too many of those magic nutritional formulae ('shed a stone with our amazing new cornflakes diet – throw away the cornflakes and just eat the box') seem automatically to assume that the human body long ago ceased all forms of natural physical movement. So instead they tell only half the story, concentrating on the need to reduce your intake of calories, rather than suggesting the other simple alternative: increasing the expenditure of calories through a controlled exercise programme.

To crash-diet clichés like 'you too can regain that lost figure' ought to be added 'as long as you're willing to starve yourself, and don't give in too often to the temptation to buy a Mars bar at times of the consequent stress'.

As an athletics coach for 20 years I have been preparing runners to get into the best possible shape for every level of competition up to and including the Olympic Games. But recently there has been a staggering increase in the number of requests for help from people who have no competitive ambitions. Instead they are people who have realised that simply chewing lettuce leaves and peeling carrots in search of the physical refurbishment they desire is soul-destroying. And, anyway, the stress they feel from being overweight is compounded by the new stress they generate by feeling forever hungry.

Women, in particular, complain that they are frustrated and perplexed; they constantly attempt endless new diets, yet seldom complete any of them. 'I've got a 'fridge full of mouldy salad, and dozens of yoghurts way past their sell-by dates,' grumbled one housewife, 'yet I'm four pounds heavier than I was a month ago. What can I do?' Empty your 'fridge before it constitutes a health hazard for a start, I suggested.

'But why is it,' she continued, 'that we see these female athletes racing round the running tracks on television looking so trim and healthy? Surely they don't exist on lettuce leaves and grapefruit juice all year?' They don't, I assured her. In fact, many of our most successful female competitive athletes of recent years have been housewives, with homes to organise, and husbands (and sometimes children) to feed. Many have full or part-time jobs: being a successful athlete doesn't release you from the need to go shopping, pay the mortgage, do the ironing, or mow the lawn.

But they don't need to go on special diets to keep

their trim figures. The exercise they get while training looks after that for them through a very simple piece of human arithmetic.

- When you eat, you take in calories.

- If you eat too much, you store the excess calories as fat.

- When you exercise, you burn up calories.

A calorie is the unit of measurement of the energy value of food, and is defined as the amount of heat required to raise one gram of water from 15°C to 16°C. However, this original calorie unit is so small that it is usable only as a term of measurement in the laboratory. So the calorific values that we use today are actually measurements made in the kilocalorie, which equals 1,000 times the value of the original calorie. In nutritional work, this is expressed as '1kcal'.

If you take in, say, 2,000 kilocalories a day, but regularly burn up 2,500 kilocalories in exercise, then clearly you will soon begin to lose weight. However, if you take in that same 2,000 kilocalories a day, but indulge in very little exercise, then much of that surplus intake will become stored fat. And day after day, week after week, month after month with little exercise means an awful lot of stored fat, which in women gathers mainly around the hips, thighs and bottom.

To be honest, it's not quite as clinically simple as that because even the most inactive of us still needs a number of kilocalories just to stay alive each day, supporting what is known as the basal metabolic rate. That keeps us breathing while we're asleep, and supplies the brain with oxygen.

Then we also need energy to support the cell activity involved in growth and the repair of damaged tissues. We need energy, too, for our most basic daily activities, even if that means merely walking from the bed to a chair.

One estimate of the average minimal calorie requirements is 1,500 kilocalories for an adult man, and 1,300 kilocalories for an adult woman. But another variable is the amount of physical work that is carried out during the day. A coal miner working hard for six hours might need 2,700 kilocalories to support that activity alone, never mind his requirements for the rest of the day. But a sedentary desk worker might find 2,000 kilocalories sufficient for the whole 24-hour day. The office-bound woman reaching out for a chocolate biscuit during her tea-break is unlikely to need the calories it contains to satisfy any nutritional need; it is more likely that it will just provide temporary relief and comfort in the face of stress or intense boredom, and add a little more padding on her hips. 'Where's it all coming from?' she will probably wonder.

We are all different, and our basic individual energy requirements differ too. The naturally thin, restless, nervy type of person may have what we could call a high metabolic rate, constantly burning up energy and rarely putting on weight. For most of the rest of us, though, it seems to be a constant battle to balance those calories.

The basically sound theory behind most diets is that if you can deliberately reduce the number of calories you consume (by maintaining a designated diet of very low calorie foods) to an amount that is less than your daily output, there will be a weight loss. However, you do not need to be Einstein to work out that if your daily expenditure of calories is low, then your intake of calories will need to be *even* lower. This eventually leads to those agonising decisions such as whether you can allow yourself one crispbread or two. What an unnecessarily miserable existence some people must have, simply because they believe there is no other way!

And trying to measure your rate of progress merely by reading the bathroom scales reflects only one part of the battle. For the benefits of becoming involved in a structured exercise programme are that it not only allows you to take in more calories while still losing weight, but also provides you with a healthier, fitter, toned up body, which dieting alone certainly cannot achieve.

Indeed, to lose weight simply through the severe dieting now engaged in by so many women in the so-called civilised world also has a number of other drawbacks. The first, as I have mentioned, is that dieting can be extremely stressful in itself. Constantly having to avoid enjoyable foods or drinks, particularly at a time of other stresses, such as exams, strained or ending relationships, financial worries, problems at work or bringing up children, can build up the frustration. In turn that frustration usually ends sooner or later by the victim succumbing to temptation and making a sudden dash to the corner shop for the comfort of chocolate. This not only greatly increases the day's intake of calories, and undoes all the good work, but also very quickly generates an associated guilt.

In more obsessed or self-disciplined individuals, the satisfaction gained from actually being able to overcome and control this natural temptation can sometimes develop into the so-called slimmer's diseases, anorexia nervosa and bulimia nervosa, which are explained more fully on pages 43–49. But the vast majority of women are forever 'dieting' unsuccessfully. Subsequently, there are very many women who view their abandonment of any calorie-controlled diet as some kind of disastrous failure or weakness. It adds little to their self-esteem. Yet such an outcome is totally unnecessary, because the odds against most people ever being able to meet the rigorous demands of the calorie-controlled diet while living a normal life are enormous. A minority might succeed (though for how long?) but I suspect the vast majority do not. I confess total sympathy with the lapsed dieter who probably spends her days munching crispbreads and apples and her nights dreaming of banana splits and chocolate gâteaux.

But trying to control weight solely through a restricted nutritional intake is an unnatural activity which should have no place in the life of any healthy adult. We all need a regular physical outlet, because the human body was designed for movement, not vegetation. Controlling weight by diet alone is like trying to repaint your broken-down car, hoping it will look better, while ignoring the need to repair the fault. And any regime which seeks merely to produce the illusion of health and fitness through a kind of starvation process is potentially dangerous.

Additionally, only the most carefully-researched diets can be effective in ensuring that the body still receives sufficient essential proteins, vitamins and minerals to maintain basic good health. A table of approximate calorific values of different foods and an indication of a minimum recommended daily intake can produce all sorts of distortions. Someone eating half a ton of raw carrots every day might theoretically be absorbing enough calories, but the lack of different nutrients would sooner or later affect their well-being.

For instance, taking in insufficient iron from the foods you do allow yourself can result in anaemia, especially in women, who lose iron during menstruation. And at best, constant dieting can still leave the individual increasingly vulnerable to infection, fatigue, lethargy and self-pity. Do you really want to be thin but miserable?

So am I suggesting that you should just be eating and drinking as much as you like, and damn the diet? Not quite, I'm afraid. Heart disease is still one of the biggest killers in the Western world, but maintaining health and fitness while controlling weight is a preventive measure which can still enable you to enjoy life more.

In this book I am not going to dictate what you can or can't eat, or produce endless recipes involving desiccated coconut and crushed grapefruit. To do so would be directing you towards a life of unalleviated stress! Instead, I am suggesting that there is the potential for much greater self-satisfaction if you assess your own food intake, and decide how you can most sensibly adjust it. I don't want people starving themselves at lunch-time when they feel like a good, solid sandwich.

I would also encourage you, though, to consider which parts of your meals really are nutritional, and which are merely comfort or habit foods. If it is part of your daily routine to have a sticky bun at 11 o'clock, you could perhaps modify your habit by replacing the bun with a piece of fruit, which would settle any genuine hunger pangs just as well. Imagine 365 sticky buns piled up alongside 365 pieces of fruit and ask yourself which you would have preferred to have eaten over the past 12 months.

The decision over whether (and what) to cut down will be yours and yours alone. For if you have reached the stage of being sufficiently concerned about your figure or well-being to read this book, you will undoubtedly already know by now what you can or cannot eat in moderation or to excess. You have probably read it all before in a dozen magazine articles.

By switching your attention from diet to exercise, I hope I will also be alerting you to several of the side-effects of exercise. First, it can be a great hunger suppressant; second, it can burn up stored calories; and third, it offers an alternative to sitting by the biscuit tin.

What I am offering is a controlled exercise plan which is totally new in its concept, but has, I suppose, been developed over the 20 years of trial and error with runners and joggers of all standards. It is based on the same coaching principles my runners have used to prepare for major international events like the Olympic Games and World and European championships. At the same time, the actual routines featured here are not designed to turn you into a world record-breaking runner. Instead, they have been specially formulated in response to the specific requirements outlined by a number of mainly inactive women between the ages of 15 and 52. These gallant ladies, who between them reflected a wide spectrum of degree of overweight, were initially assembled, and their views sought, by my wife, who had already successfully persuaded some of them to take up jogging for fitness.

Their subsequent enjoyment of the physical invigoration, and their declared frustration with a whole succession of hyped-up 'wonder' diets, led to the formulation of the activity tables. Initially, they wanted help in becoming significantly trimmer, fitter, lighter and healthier. I asked how they thought I could best help them. What *they* wanted, the consensus said, was:

1. To lose weight and to firm up, particularly in the region of the buttocks and thighs.

2. Not to have to follow yet another aimless lettuce-leaf diet plan, but instead to benefit by using a sympathetically layered exercise programme which would serve as the focus of their campaign alongside their own determination to eat more sensibly.

3. To have some definite motivational framework over a specific period (later defined as 10 weeks), which would somehow maintain their interest and encourage them to exercise even on those days when they otherwise wouldn't really feel like it. The lack of lasting motivation, they admitted, was where every other diet and exercise plan had gone adrift.

4. To have a choice of different physical activities, together with considerable flexibility as to when and where they could achieve their exercise target. This was to make allowances for uninviting dark winter evenings, thunderstorms, lack of baby-sitters, absence of training partners, work commitments, limited time availability, and enforced waits at home for the television repair man to call.

The resulting Temple Tables, the workings of which are fully explained later in the book, will, I hope, be able to fulfil these requirements for many more than the original group which acted as guinea pigs for the programme. Their experiences provided very helpful feedback on the practicalities of the tables. For a start, although they liked the points-scoring concept which rewarded each exercise, they found the original tables and scoring charts far too complicated. The result was that I simplified the system into one easier-to-follow programme for this book. They then reported on their experiences in following the plan with the tables, and you can read some of these in Chapter 6.

In developing a concept which would be helpful to the majority, I had to allow for the fact that many women still do not take part in any recreational activity, and so the introduction of exercise has to be gradual and sensible. But there is surely a huge irony in a situation where so many millions of women are desperate for help in losing weight and trimming up, yet apparently so reluctant to take part in sport or physical recreation, which would help them do just that.

Some women undoubtedly still feel, with unnecessary guilt, that there is something of a stigma attached to a woman who wants to exercise, even though hearts and lungs have no gender. So the types of activity I have incorporated offer the opportunity for the whole programme, if required, to be conducted out of sight, within four walls at home.

Alternatively, the whole exercise programme could be totally and successfully completed in public by walking in 'civvies', without anyone else knowing what you're doing. I hope, though, that most users of the tables will mix the different activities to earn their requisite scores, and be proud to do so, as well as encouraging their friends and neighbours to have a go. Apart from the immediate benefit to your own body, this attitude may help to check an unhealthy trend which is developing as we head towards the 21st century. There are already warning signs that the next generation may prove to be the least fit in history. The invention of modern transport systems, from the motor car to Concorde, and the growing and undoubted attractions to young people of television, videos and computers, are developing a largely inactive generation.

A study by a research team at Exeter University in 1989, based on a representative sample of 260 children in southern England between the ages of 11 and 15, suggested that more than 50 per cent of the girls and over one third of the boys *never* took part in physical activity equivalent to a 10-minute jog or a fast walk at four miles an hour. Only 12 per cent of the girls and 23 per cent of the boys exercised at such a level every day. And these were healthy schoolchildren, remember, not office-bound professionals. The director of the university's Physical Education Association Research Centre, Mr Neil Armstrong, observed that the study, the first of its kind in Britain, showed 'surprisingly low levels' of physical activity.

'This research suggests that many children seldom experience the intensity or duration of physical activity which is associated with prevention of coronary heart disease in adults,' he added. The research also suggested that at 13, girls were significantly less active than boys, or even than 10-year-old girls.

One of the more contradictory aspects of this is that while children are apparently taking relatively little exercise, they are also maturing earlier. For girls, taking a real interest in boys and in their own appearance may start as young as 13 or 14, at a time when puberty is beginning to wreak havoc with their hormones. The development in teenage girls of 'puppy fat', which is really just an outward sign that the body is going through its inevitable and essential change into adulthood, and their first intense concerns about getting fat begin at this time.

Self-consciousness about their changing bodies may deter girls from maintaining physical recreation, yet their introspection may be enormous. Breakfasts are skipped in the first subconscious attempts at dieting, but the physical needs of the body may prevail. Driving through any town, it is not unusual to see adolescent school-children at 8.30 in the morning swigging a can of fizzy drink and holding a half-eaten chocolate bar bought at the corner shop on their way to school.

Psychologists have shown that, whatever your age, very often unhappiness, uncertainty or stress can be briefly relieved by food. But it is usually food that your body does not actually need for nutritional purposes and it is these extra calories that show themselves in the stored fat deposits growing around your hips and thighs. The sensitivity about being overweight further increases the stress levels, and at times of high stress the temptation to eat even more for comfort is enormous. And so the vicious circle continues.

Throughout this book I have tried to spell out in detail the way you can break your way out of the downward spiral by reducing your stress level through the physical outlet of planned exercise. Finally it is *you* that has to decide: are you going to stay as you are, always putting it off until tomorrow, and then groaning when you can't get into your bikini next summer? Or are you going to get up out of your chair and finally tackle the problem realistically?

# —2—

A dozen of the world's finest women athletes were just lining up on the track in the huge Olympic stadium. There were 80,000 spectators in the stadium, and hundreds of millions of television viewers the world over, all primed for this long-awaited Olympic final. Years of training had gone into each perfectly-tuned athlete's preparation, and months of selection races and preliminary rounds. Now the moment of truth had arrived. The stadium crowd fell quiet, the runners leaned forward, and the starter raised his pistol.

Later, I asked one of the athletes what she had been thinking at that precise second. Was she considering her tactics, perhaps, or her chances of a gold medal, or realising that this was the race that would carve her name indelibly in the annals of Olympic history?

She considered carefully. 'No,' she answered finally. 'I was just wondering how big my bum looked in those shorts.'

The very idea, of course, was ridiculous. Yet it reflects a wide-reaching feminine concern. When even wafer-thin Olympic distance runners and matchstick-like model girls imagine that they see reflections of baby elephants in their wardrobe mirrors, where does that leave everyone else? It is not, after all, a problem that would have concerned the woman of the early 17th century, when the well-rounded shape, captured by Rubens, was so anxiously sought, nor the Victorian woman, with her bustled dress. But the late 20th century has yielded a whole generation to whom Eternal Happiness would be getting into a size 10 dress and still being able to breathe.

There are a great many unhappy women to whom the continuing improvement of international relations between East and West and the abolition of all nuclear weapons would mean absolutely nothing if they still could not get those damned jeans zipped up. The preoccupation with their size, particularly as it is perceived from behind, has reached epidemic proportions. The considerable majority among 3,500 women who took part in a survey for one British slimming magazine complained that their greatest single unhappiness was the size of their bottom. But only three per cent of women in the same survey were concerned about their bust.

Such surveys, reported with understandable zeal and regularity by slimming magazines, also reflect a nation in which virtually every woman from mid-teens upwards would apparently like to lose some weight. Yet those same women freely admit to a weakness for the wrong food, and take only a relatively small amount of physical exercise. It is a pattern which, unless it can be consciously and voluntarily broken, makes for constant self-defeat. Yet it is repeated in many other Western countries. It has also nurtured an enormous industry which markets hope by first spreading gentle despair.

Every woman likes to look her best, and although it is possible simply to buy over the counter most of the items needed to help her (clothes, cosmetics, hair products, jewellery), weight reduction is something that really does have to be achieved rather than purchased. There are people who would like you to believe you *can* buy it, however. The results are often disappointing.

- A massage with scented oils may be a wonderful experience, reducing stress, and relaxing muscles, which is fine in itself. *But* it won't make you lose any weight.

- A series of electrical stimulating pads may help you to tone up certain muscles if they are used often enough. *But* it won't make you lose any weight.

- Sweat-shedding garments may make you believe you are losing pounds. But you're actually only shedding water, and will drink it all back on again shortly afterwards. *And* you won't really have lost any weight.

The same marketing forces have elevated 'cellulite' into being a threat somewhat akin to the Black Death. In fact, so-called cellulite, a fashionable word introduced by a French cosmetic surgeon, is merely the fat that women accumulate around their hips and thighs. But the unnecessary reverence it receives in some quarters (particularly from those selling anti-cellulite creams) is extreme. Cellulite has come to represent something far more unpleasant than it actually is:

*Housewife*: Tell me, Doctor . . . is it serious?

*Doctor (gravely)*: I'm not certain, but I think it could be . . . it just might be . . . cellulite.

*Housewife*: Cellulite? Oh God, anything but that! (*She pauses to grasp the full significance.*) Is . . . is there a cure?

*Doctor*: Well, there's always cosmetic surgery for a couple of thousand pounds. Or special creams at £20 a jar. Or an electric massager at . . .

*Housewife*: I can't afford any of those, Doctor. Isn't there anything which comes free?

| Doctor: | Well, there is ... but I'm afraid it would involve ... exercise! (*Chord of dramatic music.*) |
| Housewife: | Exercise! (*She breaks down sobbing hysterically.*) ... |

Fortunately, one of the aims of this book is to demystify the process of becoming slimmer, trimmer and fitter. In recent years it has become exaggeratedly complicated. Are we really to believe, for instance, that over the centuries Nature has allowed women to become so uncontrollably obese that their only hope of ever becoming thinner is to purchase a vibrating belt?

It is extraordinary how much money is needlessly spent, for instance, in pursuit of the Better Bottom. Vast numbers of electric massagers, special thigh creams, and even dietary pills are bought in hope, tried in earnest, and then usually abandoned in despair.

Emma Nicholson, the MP for West Devon and Torridge, even raised the problem in Parliament in May 1989. In welcoming action from the Home Office to ban commercial slimming clinics from supplying certain habit-forming drugs as a dietary aid to their patients, she added, 'My sex, being ultra-sensitive about their shapes and sizes, are ultra-gullible in slimming.'

Yet there still remains this continual hope of one day finding the Holy Grail: a method of rapidly developing a sleeker rear which can somehow be achieved with the minimum of effort and a total disregard for physiology (and preferably one that also allows you to eat unlimited volumes of chips and chocolate). Unfortunately, that really is just a dream. And if you believe otherwise, then it is little wonder that there is no shortage of people ready to offer you gadgets and creams and to relieve you of the money which you might otherwise have spent on re-stocking your wardrobe with a new selection of a size smaller clothes.

For the enduring, healthily-refined Better Bottom is

really not achieved by the strapping on of electric pads or the rubbing in of magic oils. Nor does it cost a penny. Why should it? After all, you can never claim that your bum's too big simply because you couldn't afford a smaller one!

It is one of life's peculiarities that many of those millionairesses whose lifestyles and worldly goods you may envy would probably swap it all (well, some of it, anyway) to have a trimmer figure. But, as many ladies of substance have discovered to their intense frustration and annoyance, money cannot automatically buy a trim figure ('Hello, is that Harrods? Could you send me over a new size 10 bottom immediately, please? My present one seems to have got out of control').

The nearest thing to being able to buy slimness is obtainable through the knife of the cosmetic surgeon in what are acknowledged as sometimes risky, and always expensive, operations. In response to the demands of vanity and impatience (and the availability of substantial funds), they can vacuum away pockets of excess fat simply by making a small incision in the skin and inserting a narrow suction tube.

The best-known advertisement for cosmetic surgery is probably the American pop singer Cher, who has spent some £25,000 in recent years on such operations, including two on her buttocks at £3,000 each (operation, not buttock). However, what is rarely mentioned is that she supplements the operations by spending three hours a day exercising in her own gym, including walking two miles on a treadmill. At least Cher has now apparently appreciated that true trimming and toning comes from within. Yet many cosmetic surgery patients just allow the fat to accumulate again and then book in for another operation. Eventually, to save valuable operating time, they will probably be asked to have the traditional sites of their pockets of fat fitted with zip fasteners. Or even Velcro.

Their surgeons, of course, will need two vacuum tubes: one for the fat and the other for the money.

To those of us outside the mainstream weight-loss industry, it is bemusing to observe that this self-perpetuating routine is carried on when the answer to every weight-watcher's prayer is so simple and so obvious.

In the years I have been coaching runners my biggest problem has not been that they were too fat. Instead, it was that some of them, particularly the most successful, were becoming too thin! They had to be encouraged to eat more high carbohydrates to maintain their energy supplies, because regular exercise gobbles up the calories and reduces the fat reserves.

Your simple, no-nonsense road to a trimmer figure could not be more clearly nor directly marked than the M1 motorway. Yet some people are still tempted to meander off down country lanes and side roads, distracted by signposts promising a short-cut via 'The New All-Chip Diet' and 'Fat-Dissolving Aromatherapy Oil'. Then they wonder why their weight loss does not seem to be getting them anywhere. Yet all it needs is to switch from a daily routine which puts weight on to one which takes it off. All that is required for proof is the type of simple sum which can be found in any child's primary arithmetic book.

| Day | Calories in hand today | Calorie intake today | Calorie expenditure today | End of day total |
|-----|-----|-----|-----|-----|
| Monday | 1 unit | + 2 | − 1 | = 2 |
| Tuesday | 2 units | + 2 | − 1 | = 3 |
| Wednesday | 3 units | + 2 | − 1 | = 4 |

And so on. In other words, if you continually take in more calories than you expend, your daily fat 'stock' continually rises. But if you alter the balance, so that regular physical activity increases, then you can reverse the process:

| Day | Calories in hand today | Calorie intake today | Calorie expenditure today | End of day total |
| --- | --- | --- | --- | --- |
| Thursday | 4 | + 2 | − 3 | = 3 |
| Friday | 3 | + 2 | − 3 | = 2 |
| Saturday | 2 | + 2 | − 3 | = 1 |

Another way of reaching the same result would be to reduce the daily intake of calories, which is what happens when you 'go on a diet'. The most practical disadvantages of this are that in order to achieve significant and lasting results, the diet must be sustained for a considerable length of time. Mentally, that can be very hard, with the ever-present temptation of dropping a cream bun into the basket during a stressful shopping expedition in Tesco's with two cantankerous children quickly ending all your good intentions.

Yet the basic process of weight-loss really has no need to put its pursuers through such mental hardship. To try simply to diet weight off seems to me like trying to push a piece of rope uphill: it can be done so much more easily if someone points out a different way. By following a regular exercise programme, the number of calories which can be taken in *while* still allowing an overall weight loss is that much higher. And surely taking some exercise, even if it is only a walk round the block, cannot really be so much more of a daunting prospect than rigidly trying to abstain from food? What actually happens is this:

- Women have greater natural fat stores than men.

- They have the same access as men to a wide range of convenience foods.

- But they also have more limited opportunity (or encouragement, or access, or motivation, or all four) to take sufficient exercise to tip the balance between calories taken in and calories expended.

The surplus calories each day are therefore stored as more fat.

It is perfectly true, of course, that there are often very good reasons why women find themselves in this top-heavy calorie situation. They may be married, working, running the home, looking after the children – or all four – with constant demands from every quarter. These are just the types of stresses which make it so much easier to grab a chocolate biscuit from the tin and to sit, exhausted, in front of the television when the children have finally gone to bed. As a father of four, I have every sympathy and admiration for these unsung heroines.

If you think I'm just softening the blow for what's coming next, I am. The fact is that in terms of any sensibly progressive weight reduction programme, all these other demands have to be viewed as irrelevant. When I'm coaching international athletes, I can't go to the Olympic organisers and say, 'Excuse me, this athlete has hurt his foot, and he missed a month's training in March, and he works in a coal mine, so can he have a 10-yard start on all the others, please?'. But to overcome the practical problems, the points-scoring system I have evolved can be used indoors on a wet, windy night, or during a walk through the countryside on a sunny day. There are, I'm afraid, very few legitimate excuses as to why, whatever situation you are in, you cannot score at least some points towards your weekly target.

**Remember that losing weight is not actually a difficult process. It's just that, unfortunately, gaining weight is slightly less difficult.**

The surest way to achieving the sort of figure you want comes from within you, at no cost. It involves:

1. Motivation
2. Self-appraisal
3. Realism
4. Determination

1. **Motivation:** If you weren't to some extent already motivated to reducing your rear, you wouldn't be reading this book. But having a specific target, such as getting back into a pair of jeans you were last able to wear two years ago, or losing three inches from your hips, can help give some perspective to the size of the task, and your subsequent progress.

2. **Self-appraisal:** I am going to have to rely on you being honest about yourself when it comes to assessing the most likely causes of your expansion. If, for example, you can convince yourself that the two chocolate biscuits you consumed with your morning coffee have no real bearing on it, then we really have got an uphill struggle, haven't we?

3. **Realism:** This is a little different to self-appraisal, although it also involves recognising reality. You cannot change the body-type nature has given you (see Chapter 3), but you can make the best of it. Similarly, in your late teens there is the very real possibility that your changing hormones are more responsible for your change in shape than your diet.

4. **Determination:** I am confident that if you stick to the Temple Tables, which begin on page 79, for the prescribed 10 weeks, you will become trimmer, lighter and fitter. But only you can decide that you're going to see it through. That is where the determination comes in: yours, because you already want it to be successful, and mine, because by the time you reach page 79, I want you to want to do it!

# −3−

Before we get too involved in trying to remove fatty deposits from this key area, let's just remind ourselves exactly what makes up this particular part of the anatomy. After all, what is your bottom when it's reduced to mere muscle and bone?

It may be 'nature's well-protected back door', but it is still important to differentiate between what are its essential anatomical mechanisms and what is merely surplus blubber. After all, there is no point trying to diet or exercise away some annoying bumps which are in reality part of your pelvis! And where exactly do all these buttock muscles we are going to tone up begin and end? How many are there, what are they called, and where actually are they?

The bottom could be defined as the area behind the pelvis, which is the large basin-shaped ring of bone at the lower end of the trunk that protects the delicate organs. It also supports the vertebral column and is itself supported by the legs. Following puberty, the female pelvis usually becomes significantly wider than that of the male, in readiness for possible pregnancy, and nowhere else in the body is there such a noticeable difference in corresponding bones between the sexes. The female pelvis is roomier and shallower than that of the male, and its outlet is wider, to facilitate the passage of a baby's head when giving birth, while the thigh bone (the femur) is situated at a more acute angle than in the male.

It is unfortunate, therefore, that the pressures of fashion can become such that some women, quite unreasonably, even begin to resent or become depressed by this most natural change in their shape. Part of the reason for the distressingly blossoming hips that accompany puberty is often attributable simply to the temporary hormonal changes and the changing shape of the pelvis, and has nothing to do with diet.

## MUSCLES

The muscles in the buttocks are known as the gluteal muscles. The biggest of these is the gluteus maximus, which is broad and flat and sweeps diagonally across the buttock, connecting the pelvis with the outside of the thigh bone. It is principally this facing pair of left and right gluteus maximus muscles that help give the buttocks their characteristic shape. But that shape can soon become depressingly distorted through the accumulation of too many stored calories in the form of fat gathering, as it does in women, around the hips, thighs and bottom. The 'classic' shape can also be distorted simply by the weakness and lack of tone in the gluteus maximus muscles, caused by a lack of exercise and too much sitting. Our aim is not only to get rid of that excess flab, but also to tone up the limp buttock muscles – mere dieting won't do that for you.

Partially covered beneath the layer of the gluteus maximus are the smaller gluteus medius and minimus muscles which are of vital importance to posture. During walking or running, these muscles help to stabilise the trunk by pulling the pelvis into line with the weight-bearing limb, and make it possible for you to stand on one leg. In fact, walking and running consist of little more than alternately standing on each leg, but at different rates! If you take very little exercise, these muscles are also among those which soon become weak, lose their tone and disappear amid a sea of stored fat.

The hamstrings are a group of three long muscles at the back of the thigh, extending upwards from the back

# ANATOMY SKETCH
## REAR VIEW

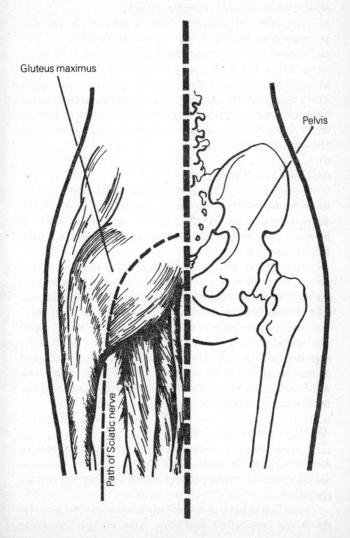

Gluteus maximus

Pelvis

Path of Sciatic nerve

of the knee to attach at the top within the buttock area. They are anchored there to a bony lump at the lower rear of the pelvis, called the ischial tuberosity (also sometimes known as the seat bone), which is actually covered by the broad gluteus maximus muscle.

The gluteal muscles are often chosen by the medical profession as the site of any intramuscular injection. This is because they offer the required opportunity to inject deep into the muscle, yet away from major nerves and arteries. Usually such injections are given in the 'upper outer quadrant' (the top right hand corner, in the case of the right buttock, to you and me) because there is even less chance of the needle touching the gluteal artery or the sciatic nerve.

## SCIATIC NERVE

The sciatic nerve itself is a long, thin nerve which emerges from either side of the spinal cord, between the lumbar vertebrae in the lower back, then extends downwards through both buttocks and the whole length of the rear of the legs.

Although we tend to think of sciatica as being a pain in the lower back, the sciatic nerve is sometimes subject to what is called 'referred pain', where the particular site of the cause of pain, such as a slipped disc, is itself pain-free, while pain may actually be felt much lower down the sciatic nerve, either in the buttock or the back of the leg. It can be a dull ache rather than a sharp pain, and whenever it is felt at the back of the thigh it is often confused, even by experienced sports physiotherapists, with a hamstring injury.

## WHICH LEAVES ... FAT

The fundamental reason why your bottom continues to become bigger in adult life is that it is simply accumulating stores of fat (sometimes called, for no good reason, cellulite).

Your bones have not suddenly filled out; your muscles have not expanded sideways. You are just carrying around unnecessary deposits of fat evolved from the excess intake of food which is not being burned up as energy. And whereas in men such excess is stored mainly around the middle, with the 'spare tyre' eventually becoming a sizeable paunch, in women nature directs the unwanted fat to the hip and thigh region.

While this book is designed to divert your pre-occupation away from severe diets, and alert it instead to the far healthier method of weight control through increased exercise, a sensible assessment of your eating habits will nevertheless make the process of trimming you up much simpler. After all, it's difficult to empty the bath while the taps are still running.

I hope, of course, that following the exercise pro-gramme will also assist you to avoid the temptation, when under stress or bored, to reach for the biscuit tin. But it's as well to be aware, in very simple terms, of which foods pose the greatest threat to undermining your new regime. The answer, as you may already have guessed, is the most tempting ones: the cream buns, the bars of chocolate, the puddings and cakes, the cream-covered gâteaux, and anything which contains a high level of sugar. These have such a high carbohydrate content that you would need to undertake an enormous amount of exercise to completely wipe out their effects. And while carbohydrates are indeed an essential part of a balanced diet, in these items they are just too concentrated to form a regular part of your daily diet if you are looking for weight control.

Calories obtained from sugar are really empty calories. Apart from energy, they give you very little towards your essential balanced diet (and contribute to tooth decay) and the brief pleasure of eating such sweet things can lead you down the wrong path. The short enjoyment will only have caused more unsightly fat to be stuffed into your hips, even if it did provide a moment of escape. Understanding the circumstances in which you succumb is the first step towards halting it.

Cutting down on fats will also help you. Using

skimmed milk instead of full fat, low fat spreads instead of butter, eating low fat cheeses (cottage cheese has much less fat than cheddar, for example) and low-fat yoghurts also means consuming less unnecessary fat. Grill rather than fry food, and remember that red meat contains far more fat than white meat. A modest proportion of foods like chicken and white fish, eggs and beans, will also ensure you receive sufficient protein, which is needed to help repair and maintain body tissues.

To replace the unhelpful foods, you could increase your intake of unrefined carbohydrates and fibre by stepping up your consumption of whole grain cereals, wholemeal flour, brown rice, wholewheat pasta and similar foods.

The more serious you are about your re-shaping, the less you will need urging to cut back on alcohol. And as one of our guinea pigs said, 'Once you start noticing the benefits of the exercise programme, you almost subconsciously begin to self-censor your dietary intake. I stopped eating sticky buns, not because I was told to, but because I began to feel so good in myself after exercise that I just didn't feel a need any more.' It's true. People who habitually eat snacks often do so because they are unhappy with themselves, and find a form of comfort from eating. A motivated exercise programme can give you a new form of self-respect where the snacking is no longer required, nor missed.


## BODY TYPES

Another consideration often overlooked in pursuit of improvements to the figure is that Nature really did intend some people to be heavier than others, and provided a wide range of different physiques. One frequently-used method of classifying these differences was developed by the American psychologist W.H. Sheldon half a century ago, and is known as Somatotyping. It recognises three basic types of physique:

- **The Endomorph:** Heavily-built, rounded shape, with a relatively high amount of body fat which increases with age. The upper arms and thighs are usually large in relation to calves and fore-arms.

- **The Mesomorph:** Well-built, broad-framed, but with large bones, high muscle mass, and a low body fat content.

- **The Ectomorph:** Slight, thin, low muscle mass and low body fat, with narrow hips, long and angular physique.

A standardised three-figure classification is achieved by crediting a score on a scale of 1 to 7, reflecting the degree to which the subject displays the characteristics of each of the three basic types. Thus, an extreme meso-morph would be categorised as 1-7-1, while someone exhibiting an equal balance between all three types would be recorded as 4-4-4. Sadly for those who would like to try, it is simply not possible to change these natural characteristics. There are millions of women who would love to be extreme ectomorphs to fit in well with the current trends in fashion, but nature takes no notice of fashion; only of preserving the species.

In fact, within the normal range of men and women, discounting excessive obesity or thinness, natural heights may vary by up to 30 per cent, and natural weights by up to 60 per cent. So while you can become a slimmer, fitter version of your natural body type, a true endomorph can never, even with the severest of diets, become a true ectomorph – only a very hungry endomorph!

# —4—

## PUBERTY

For many women, the problem of weight is a haunting shadow which has pursued them relentlessly from their mid-teens. Before that they may have been lively, active girls whose dietary lifeline consisted of Mars bars, crisps and fizzy drinks, with no apparent effect on their weight. But later, during and after puberty, it can be hard for them to accept that these enjoyable and convenient food items are actually betraying them, after years of consumer loyalty, by contributing to the problems now beginning to stare them in the face from the mirror. But they are by no means solely to blame. Nature must accept its share of guilt, too.

The process of change actually begins about four years before a girl experiences her first period (the menarche), which occurs on average around the age of 13 or 14. So the mechanism which leads to the changes signalled by the onset of menstruation starts around the age of 9 or 10. Gradually, and at first almost imperceptibly, the pelvis, previously of the same proportions as that of a boy, begins to broaden, and fat deposition starts.

At the same time, a gland in the brain, the hypothalamus, begins secreting 'releasing hormones', one of which, the growth hormone, sets off a growth spurt which is particularly noticeable during its first two years as the girl's height increases relatively rapidly. Around the age of 12 a further releasing hormone, the gonadotrophin-releasing hormone, is secreted by the pituitary gland, and this begins the sequence of events leading to the production by the girl's ovaries of the principal female sex hormone, oestrogen.

It is oestrogen that stimulates the growth of the breasts and nipples, the oviducts, the uterus and the vagina. It also stimulates fat to be deposited on the hips, a process which becomes even more marked and noticeable around the age range of 15 to 17. Yet it cannot be stressed too often that this is a perfectly normal pattern; to change a girl into a mature woman and prepare her for eventual motherhood, to perpetuate the species through reproduction, is Nature's aim.

However, the pure natural growth may be masked by the relatively dramatic effects of the increasing fat depositions around the hips, thighs and bottom. This is sometimes known as puppy fat, but it has nothing to do with young dogs. It is simply fat.

But why does it seem to spread so rapidly? The oestrogen that stimulates the fat deposition needs to have some fat to deposit, and this is where the crisps and chocolate come in. From having slipped through the net, so to speak, in childhood, the high-calorie foods have now become prime culprits. Unfortunately, the realisation of this coincides with a particularly difficult emotional time during adolescence. The mid-teens are the turmoil years, in which every type of value is being questioned, sexuality is explored, relationships are being sought, developed, sometimes painfully ended, or (even more painfully) proving elusive even to begin. School or college examinations loom large. Teenage social pressures to dress, look and act in a way that is acceptable to the inner circle may be stifling.

Priorities which may be baffling to the adult world find their own order. Winning a place at Cambridge University may seem of very little moment to a 17-year-old girl when her boyfriend didn't ring last night although he'd promised. And, with all these other things whirring around her head, the last thing she needs today is to find that she can no longer get into her favourite jeans either.

At such moments of depression, the temptation of 'comfort foods' rears its head. This is where the excess flab really comes from: not food to relieve genuine hunger pangs, but food taken to try to relieve stress or unhappiness, or to provide solace. Or food taken simply through habit.

In such circumstances, then, part of the way to controlling weight is to assess honestly how much of your calorific intake is actually consumed through (a) depression, or (b) habit.

Because we are all different, there are people who put on weight very easily, and those who can burn up calories very quickly. But very rarely is excess weight genuinely due to that old excuse 'trouble with her glands'. At the same time, not every overweight youngster has necessarily become so by being depressed or unhappy. But the problem can quickly become magnified if school friends pick on them (as school friends do), with the result that they do *become* depressed and unhappy, and perhaps start eating for comfort. Then it is a problem which has almost created itself, and may be difficult to break. Even harder to break, though, is an obsessional desire to be thin.

## ANOREXIA NERVOSA

A problem that often develops from the trauma of puberty is the high incidence among teenagers of the condition known as anorexia nervosa, sometimes referred to as the 'slimmer's disease'. In fact, it is not a physical disease at all, but rather an obsession with slimness, which manifests itself as a constant desire to lose weight, or at least as a perpetual fear of putting on weight.

'So what's new?' you might ask. Well, the anorexic girl is actually an extremely successful weight-loser. Far more successful than you or me. Too successful, in fact. Her body not only goes through a stage of reaching its 'ideal' state, but then carries on losing weight, because the girl herself is never satisfied that she has reached a desirable weight. So losing more weight, and being able to demonstrate her mental strength to herself by avoiding food whenever possible, becomes an obsession.

As she reduces food intake to an inadequate level, in due course a number of physical side effects occur. Her skin becomes rough and dry; nails become cracked, ridged and easily broken because of a dietary deficiency of protein, vitamins and calcium. She becomes subject to dizziness, as a result of low blood pressure. Her resistance to infection is low, and recovery from illness is slow.

To continue with an inadequate diet will cause more dramatic symptoms, including the appearance of soft, downy hair on her back, face and arms; the cessation of menstrual periods (known as secondary amenorrhoea – if she has never menstruated, a delay in their onset is known as primary amenorrhoea); and restless sleep, hyperactivity and obsession with exercise. One possible parallel to this last symptom has been suggested by scientists who note that a hungry animal rarely sleeps, but continues to prowl in the night in search of food.

In other words, the body does not welcome the inadequate intake of food at all. In extreme cases of anorexia, the girl may even reach an advanced state of malnutrition requiring hospitalisation, and still be unable to bring herself to eat anything, even though her very life may be at risk. In a disturbing number of examples of the frightening ability of the determined mind to take over the body, the eventual result is fatal. Surely there can be few more tragic circumstances than a healthy young girl becoming so totally obsessed with remaining thin that its pursuit brings a needlessly premature end to her life.

## WHO IS AT RISK?

The classic candidate for anorexia is the academically bright introvert who may be feeling real or imaginary pressure from family or teachers to reach outstanding levels of achievement. These pressures may make her feel that she has no control over her own life, and that by rigidly controlling her diet and body she manages to exert some control over herself.

Another widely noted cause of anorexia in adolescents appears to be a subconscious rebuttal of the approach of adulthood. This often proves to be linked with a happy childhood that has been prematurely ended by the separation or divorce of the girl's parents, or of open marital strife between them. Some psychologists have suggested that in such cases the subsequent onset of anorexia reflects an almost desperate attempt by the young woman to remain a small girl, as when life was so much happier. She sees the pubertal changes in her body as an end of her links with that enjoyable childhood, and tries to hold back nature's clock.

Intriguingly, this appears to happen primarily with females, but some research has indicated that the recent fitness boom among males around their 40s is the result of an equivalent type of obsession with holding back the march of time. Whereas most adolescent males can hardly wait to become adult, whatever their family background, their own type of superficial body changes at around the age of 40 (thickening waistline, thinning, greying hair) seems to sound the sort of alarm bells which have led to so many thousands taking up marathon running, or at least jogging round the park.

For females, however, the battle for trimness seems to begin with puberty and for many millions never really ends. One physiologist noted: 'The difference between the average woman and an anorexic is that although they are both constantly on diets, the anorexic has the extra determination to be successful.' But, as we have seen, that determination can actually be a dangerous attribute. In recent years, there has been an increase in eating disorders among female participants in sports such as ice-skating and gymnastics, in which the need for an aesthetically pleasing appearance is sometimes as great as that for technical skill.

Similarly, although even female Olympic athletes are as concerned as the next woman about their shape, the recent development of competitive opportunities in the sport, which now allows women to run endurance races up to, and beyond, the 26-mile marathon, have also highlighted cases of anorexia among promising young athletes. In distance races, a light frame and low body fat content is advantageous. However, it is quite possible that some of these athletes had a sufficiently intense personality to have become anorexic even if they had not taken up distance running.

## SYMPTOMS

The following symptoms may indicate dietary deficiency:

- Skin becoming rough and dry, nails becoming cracked, ridged and easily broken, due to deficiency in protein, vitamins and calcium.

- Constipation, due to inadequate dietary intake of fibre.

- Oedema (retention of body fluid) may be noticed, particularly as puffiness around legs and ankles, and may be due to lack of protein.

- Dizziness, particularly when changing position, as a result of low blood pressure.

- Weakness, which may come on suddenly, due to inadequate calorie intake.

- Slow recovery from illness.

The following additional symptoms are suggestive of anorexia nervosa:

- Continuing weight loss.

- Increasing skeletal appearance: protusion of shoulder blades, backbone, bones at hips and buttocks. Sitting for any length of time on a hard surface becomes uncomfortable.

- Regular self-weighing.

- Disturbed body image (complaining of feeling 'fat' even when emaciated).

- Hyperactivity, and obsession with exercise.

- Restless sleep and early waking.

- Cessation of periods (amenorrhoea).

- Bluish-mauve colouring at extremities, which could also be cold to the touch (acrocyanosis).

- Appearance of fine, downy hair on back, arms and legs.

- Abuse of laxatives and diuretics.

- Loner behaviour and insistence that, despite displaying many of the above symptoms, all is well.

## BULIMIA NERVOSA

Bulimia nervosa is a clinically separate condition to anorexia, although some women show signs of both simultaneously. Bulimia also revolves around an obsession with food and weight. The bulimia sufferer, or bulimic, tries desperately hard to control her weight but suffers periodic outbreaks of 'binge' eating in which she is overwhelmed by a desire to gorge a large amount of high carbohydrate food. The next stage, in her guilt or disgust at this bingeing, is to privately vomit back the food before it has been digested, and this compulsive cycle of dieting, gorging and regurgitating can be as difficult to break as that of anorexia.

Bulimia can be even more difficult to detect than anorexia, because its sufferers tend to be closer to normal weight than those of anorexia. Whereas an anorexic is likely to be quiet and introverted, the bulimic may well be extrovert, outgoing and cheerful (although inwardly very unhappy). After an apparently normal meal, the bulimic may briefly excuse herself from the table, and then secretly rid herself of the undigested food in the toilet by self-induced vomiting. Then she will rejoin the table as though nothing has happened. Warning signs include:

- General obsession with food and weight.

- Unusually frequent visits to bathroom or toilet after or between meals to 'wash my hair' or 'take a quick shower'.

- Traces of vomit in toilet or bathroom.

- Poor condition of sufferer's teeth (the acidic action of vomiting erodes tooth enamel and decay follows).

- Disappearance of food from cupboards and refrigerator.

- Fluctuations in weight over short periods of time.

- Sufferer is often short of money, having spent it on food for clandestine consumption.

- Frequent self-weighing.

- Unexplained cake, biscuit and sweet wrappings around the house (under pillows, mattress, chairs etc.)

- Lack of interest in social activities, preference to stay at home.

- Staying up alone late at night, often for further binge/purge.

- Habit developing of short, impromptu walks (in direction of food shops).

The first and most important step towards recovery for the anorexic or bulimic is to admit that there is a problem. Once they have shared their problem, even confidentially, their world may never seem quite so lonely again.

The sufferer's GP will normally be able to refer them if necessary for specialist treatment. But some anorexics and bulimics steadfastly refuse medical assistance, and it cannot be forced upon them. For them, making contact with a sympathetic self-help group may be the answer.

Many anorexics, however, still remain too shy and introverted even to visit a doctor or to approach a self-help group such as the Eating Disorders Association. For them, reading some of the growing number of books on the subject may help them to gain a perspective on their problem and, eventually, to overcome it. Reaching the ideal shape, fitness and health is not always a question of slimming down, but the end result is worth the effort.

# −5−

Before we come to the tables themselves, let's consider the basic requirements of the various points-scoring activities. There are four different ways of scoring points: by jogging, walking, performing exercises or performing isometric exercises (known here as isocises).

Many people undertaking this programme may be tackling several of these physical activities, possibly even all of them, for the first time. I hope that the standards I have set reflect this. But let's look at each in turn.

## JOGGING

A jog is a slow, steady, controlled, comfortable run, so the first necessity is to forget completely your schoolday experiences of being vociferously urged by PE teachers to run faster on a bumpy grass track or on an enforced cross-country.

Jogging is a far more enjoyable, relaxed activity than that, and yet it is one to which, unfortunately, children are rarely introduced at school. As an activity it offers enormous physical benefits to the growing (as well as to the overgrown!) body.

Sadly, the more common and miserable school experience of having to force lungs and muscles to continue at a level of output for which they have not been properly conditioned turns many youngsters away from physical exercise for life. Yet, as a coach, I would never dream of asking even an Olympic champion to run at the degree of effort often demanded of untrained schoolchildren until they had completed a sufficient background of steady, comfortable running in the preceding weeks.

That conditioning starts with jogging and, if you have never jogged before, prepare to banish all your preconceptions about how hard it is. It isn't. The only difficult part is getting people simply to try it in the first place.

### How do you start?

Well, what you *don't* do is to rush out of the front door and off down the road as far and as fast as possible until you collapse in an exhausted heap. It's much gentler than that. Some people do prefer to start jogging as far as possible on the first day, and then gradually increase the distance on subsequent outings. But a much easier way of building up to a reasonable distance (and therefore points score) is to start by alternating a series of short walks and jogs, using a footpath in the local park or recreation ground.

From your chosen starting point walk for, say, 30 seconds, and then break into a slow jog for 20 seconds. Then walk again for 30 seconds to recover, jog for another 20 seconds, and so on. The pace of the jog itself should at first be only slightly faster than the walk. And if you want a definition of the crucial difference between walking and jogging, it is that while walking you always have at least one foot on the ground, whereas in jogging both feet leave the ground momentarily on every stride.

On your first attempt, a total of 10 minutes spent alternately walking and jogging can prove quite tiring, yet exhilarating. But you have to resist any tendency to jog too quickly, because the main aim is to bring about a gradual conditioning of the cardiovascular system, helping your heart and lungs to improve their efficiency in processing and transporting oxygen from the air to your muscles. The demand increases at the time of a growing physical need, in this case brought about by jogging.

If it has been some years since they were last called upon to perform what is, after all, their perfectly normal function, they will need to be gently re-introduced to it. And as they get back into practice, like any rusty pianist, they will soon begin to improve through repetition. The longer they have been neglected, the longer it may take to get them back to their prime condition. But improvement will start from day one! The moment you start jogging you have taken, with the very first steps, your path back to achieving fitness and your rate of calorie expenditure will have increased.

### Next steps

As you become fitter day by day the next stage is to cut down the length of the walks on your outings and increase the duration of the jogging phases. For example, if you were walking for 30 seconds and jogging for 20, after three days you should be able to jog for 30 seconds and reduce the walks in between to 20 seconds.

Gradually, you will be able to jog at the same pace for longer, and you'll find that the walking recoveries become less and less essential. Within 10 days you should be able to dispense with them altogether, and jog continuously for 5-10 minutes at the same comfortable pace without stopping. Once you have reached that level, your progress will gather further momentum as your muscles and lungs quickly become adapted to the requirements you are making.

How do you know if you are jogging too fast? The most effective self-check is the 'conversation test'. This means that if you are becoming too short of breath to be able to hold a conversation with someone else jogging at the same pace, then you are going too quickly and will need to slow down until you can. You do not *need* to be gasping for air for the exercise to be doing you good.

Admittedly, the training of advanced competitive runners does involve a degree of flat-out, lung-draining runs. But that is only because the runners concerned will already have reached such a high level of basic fitness over a period of some years that the best way to induce further progress in them is to simulate the body performing as it does in a race. The body is very good at adapting to what you ask it to do. After all, that is the whole point of training.

So while your conversational-paced jogging alongside the council's neatly maintained rose bushes in the local park may seem a world away from Steve Cram training for the Olympic 1500 metres final, you are both actually working on precisely the same principle. In your case, every step you jog is helping to improve your circulation, strengthening your heart, lungs and muscles, firming you up and trimming you down!

### What do you wear?

Virtually anything, but a tracksuit or leisure suit, worn with a T-shirt, is ideal. Many women now wear them most of the day anyway, purely for comfort. But jeans are not very practical, because they restrict physical movement. A pair of training shoes, which need not be very expensive, are a wise investment, because their cushioning will reduce jarring in the legs and allow you to jog with a natural action.

Specially-designed sports bras are now widely available. They are stretchy and seam-free, and some have the added advantage of straps which join together at the back so they don't fall off your shoulders. For women who are generously endowed, and somewhat self-conscious of boob-swing, some experienced runners have discovered that wearing a second bra can make a substantial difference while jogging or running.

If you jog at night, make sure you are wearing white, orange or other light-coloured outer clothing, so that motorists can see you crossing roads. Navy blue and black jogging kit should be kept for daylight hours.

### What about jogging style?

Everyone has a natural jogging or running action, and there is no need to try to change it. But staying relaxed in the upper body, with shoulders and arms free of tension, is important so that you are able to breathe efficiently and economically. Your legs do the work, and the rest of you has little choice but to follow!

## *Can you jog with your friends?*

Jogging in a group often adds to the enjoyment of the exercise and as you become fitter, and can jog further, it helps the miles pass more quickly. However, try to ensure that your friends are of a similar level of fitness to you, because there is nothing more dispiriting than being unable to keep up, or having to jog too fast (remember the 'conversation test'). Sometimes it may be better to jog on your own, or with just one friend, so that you can keep your own progress steady.

It's also sad, but these days necessary, to have to mention the need for vigilance if you are a woman jogging alone. For that reason, try to vary your routes and jogging days. Never use a personal stereo while jogging either. It cuts you off from the world in a most hazardous fashion, including masking the sound of approaching traffic.

## *Any other considerations?*

It can be quite uncomfortable to try to jog too soon after eating: you should aim to leave at least two hours before jogging (or three after a big meal). Apart from the discomfort of the food inside you, the body will have sent blood to the stomach to help the digestive process and if it is suddenly required to divert some of that blood to the muscles to aid exercise, indigestion may result.

## WALKING

Most people think they walk much further each day than they actually do. But the beneficial effects of walking, and the simplicity with which it can earn you points, should not be overlooked.

One of the advantages of walking as a physical exercise is the vast range of circumstances in which you can combine a walk (perhaps taking a roundabout route) with an essential task, like walking to the shops or to the station, or walking to see a friend. Unlike jogging, you can take a pushchair when you walk, and you don't arrive hot and sweaty at the other end. Even a husband or boyfriend who isn't into jogging might be persuaded to walk with you.

Because it is a less vigorous form of exercise than jogging, you don't score quite so many points on the Temple Tables for the equivalent time spent walking. But then you may be inclined to go walking for a longer period than you would have jogged, and end up with the same points anyway; or more.

Even for the keen jogger, there may be days when a long walk may seem more attractive than jogging. A chance to think, and the opportunity to enjoy some time and space when everything else seems to be closing in on you, are part of the attraction too. You don't need much in the way of special clothing or equipment either, although a good pair of shoes is essential. You won't get very far in high heels.

In the USA walking has succeeded the running boom in terms of popularity, because it is something in which the whole family can participate together.

## EXERCISES

Each of the six chosen exercises in the programme is geared particularly to strengthening and de-flabbing the muscles in the buttock region. For while it is true that it is not possible to isolate particular parts of the body for weight loss (apart from the liposuction method outlined on page 27), in women any substantial weight loss will be clearly reflected in this area anyway, so toning and strengthening the muscles there in preparation for the new slim you is very important.

One of the attractions of performing a series of exercises as part of that trimming programme is the opportunity to do them whenever and wherever you wish. Some of our guinea pigs undertook the exercises in everyday clothes, squeezing the routine into a spare few minutes between other commitments. But others preferred to change into a leotard or tracksuit. Either approach is acceptable, just as long as it fits in with your available time. After all, your body doesn't know whether it is wearing a leotard or a Laura Ashley dress; only that it is being asked to perform exercises, and to adapt accordingly to those demands.

These are the exercises, illustrated in the picture section, which form this part of the programme.

## 1. Apple crush
Lie on your back on the floor, with your knees bent, and your feet placed about 10–12 inches apart and flat on the floor.

Now squeeze your buttocks hard together, then lift your hips and lower back two inches off the floor, while ensuring that your mid-back remains on the floor. Hold this position for 10 seconds (or a count of 10), then lower slowly to the floor. Recover for 10 seconds before repeating.

Number of repetitions: 6.

## 2. Kneeling squat
Kneel on the floor, remaining upright from the knees, with your arms straight out in front of you.

Now slowly lower your buttocks to the floor, keeping your body straight, until they lightly touch your heels. Hold this position for 10 seconds (or a count of 10), then slowly return to the upright kneeling position. Recover for 10 seconds before repeating.

Number of repetitions: 4.

## 3. Hippy hippy raise
Sit on the floor, with your legs straight out in front of you, feet together, and hands behind you.

Now raise your body from the floor, resting on your palms and heels, and push your hips towards the ceiling. Hold the position for 10 seconds, then lower to the floor again. Recover for 10 seconds before repeating.

Number of repetitions: 5.

### 4. Pelvic rock

Kneel on the floor, with the palms of your hands flat on the floor in front of you, and your tummy and back relaxed.

Now lift your back into a rounded arc, while pulling your pelvis forward by contracting your stomach and buttock muscles. Hold this position for 10 seconds, then relax and recover for 10 seconds before repeating.

Number of repetitions: 6.

### 5. Bottom walk

Sit on the floor, with your arms folded and your legs straight out in front of you. Then 'walk' across the room on your bottom, using only the buttock muscles. Return in a backward direction to the starting point. (NB: If this exercise becomes too easy, stretch your arms in front of you.)

Number of repetitions: 2.

### 6. Gluteal stretch

More of a relaxation than an exercise: Kneel on the floor, with your knees folded up to your chest, while resting on your palms and forearms, so that your buttock muscles are fully stretched. Once in this position, hold for 20 seconds, then stand. Wait for 20 seconds before repeating.

Number of repetitions: 3.

### ISOCISES

Isometric exercises (referred to in this book as isocises) are different from ordinary exercises because they involve no physical movement. Instead, they rely on a series of short, repeated, static contractions of the muscle to improve its strength and conditioning. Again, the four isocises selected for the programme were those which had particular relevance to the buttock area.

Believe it or not, isometrics have their origins in laboratory experiments with a frog at Springfield College, Massachusetts in the 1920s. One of the frog's legs was immobilised, but then unbound at fixed intervals. Each time it was tested the immobilised leg proved stronger than before (and much stronger than the free leg) because the frog had to use the whole muscle to move it, whereas it needed to use only part of the muscle to move its free leg.

Laboratory experiments in isometrics were performed on over 5,000 people by Dr E.A. Mueller in Germany in the 1950s. In one, a man's arm was completely immobilised, apart from a brief spell once a day when it was freed long enough for him to perform a single isometric contraction lasting six seconds. That brief exercise proved long enough for it to become stronger than his free arm, which he had been using normally.

As a result, it was thought for some years that to achieve maximum improvement in strength with this method, isometric contractions needed to be held only once, for six seconds' duration. But following experiments in the 1960s, that view was revised to a need for 5–10 repetitions, held for 5 seconds each, on five days a week, to reach optimal improvement. The regularity is also crucial in reaping the benefits of isocises. One session performed only once a week is now estimated to achieve less than half the improvement of sessions repeated daily.

Part of the success of the tables depends on their offering you the choice of different activities to dovetail with your other commitments. Isometric exercises are particularly valuable in this respect, and some of the isocises in this book can even be performed at an office desk or at a bus stop without anyone nearby even realising what you are doing!

It is important, however, that you maintain normal breathing when performing each isocise. The natural tendency is to hold your breath for each 5-second muscular contraction, but that is quite unnecessary. It could even be dangerous for anyone who suffers from hypertension because each exercise also creates a rise in blood pressure, which is immediately reduced when the tension has been released.

These are the isometric exercises in which conditioning is obtained by providing a maximum contraction for 5 seconds. You will need to be near a solid wall, and have a kitchen or office chair available, to perform all four. The isocises are illustrated in the picture section.

### 1. Ankle press
Sit on the floor, with your legs straight out in front of you. Place the back of your left ankle on top of the front of your right ankle.

Now try to raise your right ankle, while continuing to hold it down with the left. Remember to breathe normally, and hold the position for 5 seconds (or a count of 5). Change ankles, and repeat.

Number of repetitions: 5 on each ankle.

### 2. Demolition shove
Stand facing a wall, about 18–24 inches away from it. Lean on it with palms flat against the wall at chin height, 12 inches apart. Your elbows should be slightly bent, and your feet flat on the ground.

Now press hard against the wall for 5 seconds, breathing normally. You should be able to feel the muscles in your arms, shoulders, back, thighs, calves and buttocks tighten. Relax for 10 seconds, then repeat.

Number of repetitions: 5.

### 3. Knot knock kneed
Sit on a chair, and place your hands on the outside of your knees. Push inwards with your hands, while simultaneously pushing outwards with your knees. Breathe normally, and hold the position for 5 seconds. Relax for 10 seconds, and then repeat.

Number of repetitions: 8.

### 4. Leg lifter
Sit on a chair, and grip a waste paper basket, foot stool or similar object between your ankles. Then raise it, with

**Exercise 1:** Apple Crush. From the starting position (fig. 1), lift into the 'squeeze' position (fig. 2), and hold it for 10 seconds before returning slowly to the starting position.

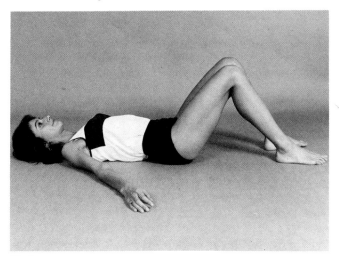

*Fig. 1*

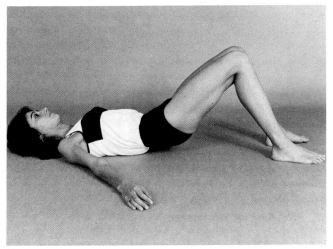

*Fig. 2*

**Exercise 2:** Kneeling Squat. From the upright kneeling position (fig. 3), slowly lower buttocks to lightly touch heels (fig. 4).

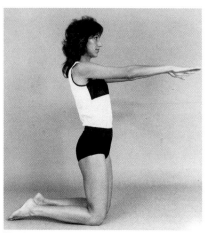

*Fig. 3*

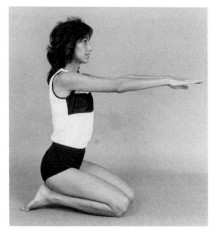

*Fig. 4*

**Exercise 3:** Hippy Hippy Raise. From relaxed starting position (fig. 5), push hips towards the ceiling (fig. 6) and hold for 10 seconds before slowly lowering to floor.

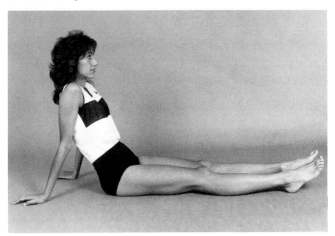

*Fig. 5*

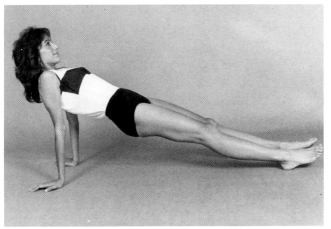

*Fig. 6*

**Exercise 4:** Pelvic Rock. From kneeling position (fig. 7), raise your back into a rounded arc (fig. 8) and hold for 10 seconds.

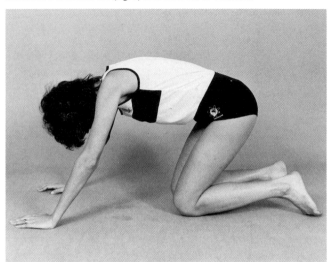

*Fig. 7*

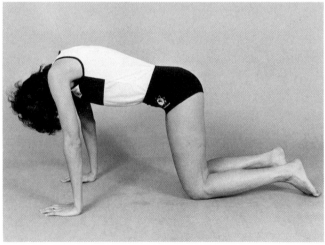

*Fig. 8*

**Exercise 5:** Bottom Walk. With arms folded, 'walk' on alternate buttocks across the room (figs. 9 and 10).

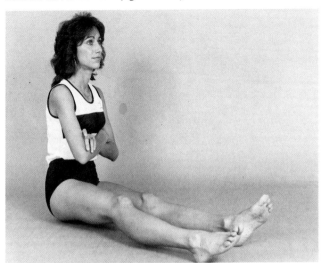

*Fig. 9*

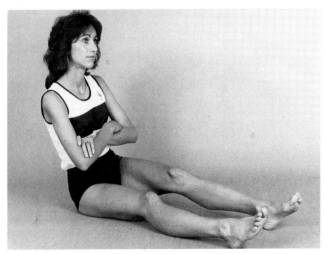

*Fig. 10*

**Exercise 6:** Gluteal Stretch (fig. 11). Fold knees to chest in a relaxed position, fully stretching the gluteal muscles of the bottom, and hold for 20 seconds at a time.

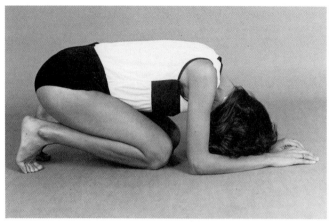

*Fig. 11*

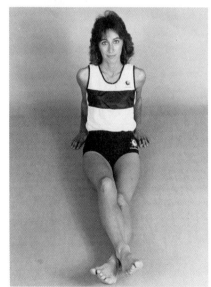

**Isocise 1:** Ankle Press (fig. 12). Try to raise one ankle while holding it down with the other.

*Fig. 12*

**Isocise 2:** Demolition Shove. From the starting position leaning against a wall (fig. 13), bend the elbows and press hard against the wall (fig. 14).

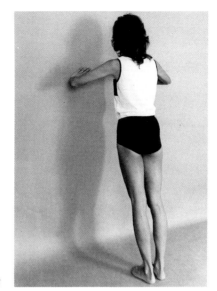

*Fig. 13*

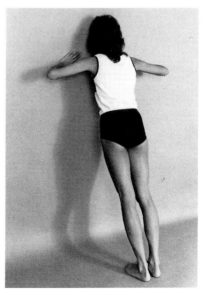

*Fig. 14*

**Isocise 3:** Knot Knock Kneed. Sit on a chair, pushing your knees inwards while resisting the force (fig. 15).

*Fig. 16*

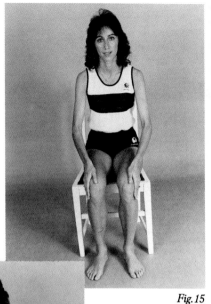

*Fig. 15*

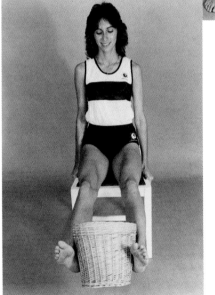

**Isocise 4:** Leg Lifter. Lift an object, such as a waste-paper basket, with your feet and hold it static by tensing the buttock muscles (fig. 16).

your legs fully extended and parallel to the ground. Hold this position static for five seconds, by tensing your buttock muscles. Remember to breathe normally. Relax for 20 seconds, and then repeat.

Number of repetitions: 5.

## OTHER ACTIVITIES

I have been repeatedly asked whether other physical activities, like swimming, cycling, squash and ice-skating, can count towards the points scoring. My initial reaction was to say no, because the simplicity of the tables was deliberate, to allow anyone to attain a new level of fitness at virtually no cost. None of the proposed activities need a partner or teammate (such as in tennis, netball, squash or hockey), nor is there any requirement to gain access to swimming pools, bicycles, or skating rinks.

However, there is no doubt that engaging in other physical activities like those I have mentioned does play its part in improving condition and fitness, and it seems unfair not to acknowledge that. I would therefore allow a score of 1 point for each continuous minute of genuine activity in those recreations. But please note that this offer does not apply to non-active sports like snooker, darts, archery, chess or angling!

## RECOVERY

Achieving progress in fitness and conditioning means finding a happy medium. If you don't put in enough time and dedication, there will be only a small gain. But, similarly, if you put in too much too soon it can also have a negative effect. As an extreme example, if you tried to exercise 20 hours a day, clearly you would soon expect to collapse with exhaustion. No one in their right mind would go that far, but sometimes genuine enthusiasm is such that too much is undertaken. Olympic runners, for example, are the world's worst for resting. If they have to take a day off with a cold or slight injury, they are usually convinced that in that idle 24 hours all the fitness they have built up in 10 or 12 years will have mysteriously vanished! And an athlete with a more serious injury can be worse than a caged tiger, fretting and panicking.

Yet very often an athlete who has been forced to rest by injury or illness comes back to competition far better than he expected. The reason, I am convinced, is because he had to give his body the rest it so badly needed to recover from the effects of hard training, and which he would never allow it voluntarily. That is why you should attempt the weekly points totals in strict sequence. Allow yourself the full ten weeks to reach 1,000 points, with the weekly gain of 100 points, rather than trying to reach Week 7's total in the third week. A steady increase in volume of exercise is far more effective than rushing it in a shorter time. It also forms a far more solid base, enabling you to maintain your newly-improved body more easily.

There are valid medical reasons for not cramming too great an increase of exercise into one week. The inevitable fatigue may reduce your resistance to infection, or you might even sustain some form of 'overuse' injury. This is the type of injury which afflicts obsessive sportsmen, caused not by sudden exertion or physical accident but simply by the sheer repetition of an exercise with insufficient recovery. Tennis elbow is an example.

For most people, though, even maintaining the weekly increase may prove enough of a challenge, and here are some tips which will help you through it. While limited time may dictate that after exercise on some days of the week you may have to freshen up with just a rapid shower or quick dip in the bath, try to enjoy at least one long, self-pampering soak each week in a bubbly, scented bath. You could even promise yourself that luxury as a reward for reaching each of the weekly points totals.

Massage is now returning to popularity as a way of restoring weary muscles and speeding recovery from sustained exercise. You can book a professional massage at many health clubs now, and it is still widely used by many physiotherapists (despite their armoury of electrical treatments) as an effective method of treating certain types of injury. But massage as a relaxing, regenerative treatment can still be effectively given by a friend or partner.

The key to progress and improvement, whether you are an Olympic athlete or just trying to restore your body, is to work hard and recover well in between.

# –6–

Before I finalised the tables, a number of 'guinea pig' volunteers tested the system. I was already perfectly confident that, on their own, the various activities and exercises could not fail to have a beneficial long-term effect unless too many sessions were skipped, forgotten, or otherwise irretrievably lost. But I wanted to be sure that the system was comprehensible and motivational, because if the tables were followed virtually to the letter, then human physiology would quickly adapt to improvement.

In the past when anyone has grumbled that they have been following a particular 'lose 10 pounds in a month' diet, or get-fit-quick campaign, and that it hasn't worked, it has usually transpired that they didn't actually follow it quite as precisely as originally recommended. So the problem in satisfying the communal desire to become thinner, fitter and healthier is *not* that there is anything basically wrong with the dietary advice, recipes and exercise programmes being offered. Instead, the weak link is more likely to be the user's constantly changing moods and levels of motivation over the necessarily extended period required for the regime to be effective.

On day one you may well be primed for action, dressed in your tracksuit and taking a surprised Fido for an elongated walk by 7.30 am. But if by day four, you are still in your dressing-gown at lunch-time, watching 'Neighbours' with a large piece of cake in your hand, then your major problem is the one shared by millions of others worldwide. It's the 'I did it yesterday, and I promise I'll do it tomorrow, but today's a day off' syndrome. Progress grinds to a halt because, however well intentioned you are, it's always today and never tomorrow! What I have tried to do, then, is produce a system which supplies you with the necessary motivation not to leave it until tomorrow. By setting you a points target which is attainable, but only if you keep yourself in hand and don't leave too much until another day, I hope to help you over the vagueness of exercise programmes which suggest 'do six of these toe-touches' every day, but offer no further incentive other than that it will do you good.

It also undermines most of the excuses you can throw at me, because at any time of the day or night, anywhere in the world, even sitting in an aeroplane half-way across the North Pole, you can score points. If it's pouring with rain and you've just had your hair done, then you can score your points from the exercises, performed on your lounge carpet. If you've just started your period and feel too yukky for anything too active, then you can still score your points from a steady walk round the block or in the park; it may even help you feel better, too. If you have a blistered foot, then score your points from the exercises or isocises. Somehow, some way, keep up with the points. Any physical, mental or social obstruction can be overcome in pursuit of those points if you really want to be that thinner, fitter person.

The only acceptable reason for not fulfilling the demands is genuine illness, including that stage of 'flu at which your whole body aches and you break into sweat. At such times, rest is better and will speed recovery. But pure laziness does not count as an illness!

Here now are some of the observations of the guinea pigs, whose help I gratefully acknowledge, because they told me when they thought the tables were too complicated, loaded, or otherwise unfair. Their observations helped shape the tables into their final form, and to decide the precise contents of the exercises and isocises.

### Nicola, 25, primary school teacher:

'I got married a year ago, and the change in my daily routine meant that I started to put on some weight. Previously, I had walked a mile every morning from my parents' house to meet a colleague who gave me a lift in her car, and I walked back in the evening. But when I got married, I started to drive to school in my husband's car, and didn't walk anywhere. So, whereas previously I had been walking two miles a day, or 10 miles a week which, even allowing for school holidays, added up to 400 miles of walking a year, suddenly I wasn't doing it any more.

'When I got home in the evening, I would just slump in a chair because I was tired from standing all day, and general stress, although I had not actually taken any real exercise. I felt very lazy, and I wasn't happy with myself, but I lacked an incentive to do anything about it. The tables added a whole new part to the day. They gave me the motivation to go out, take some exercise, and then be able to sit down for the evening with a much clearer conscience! Having a target to aim for was very helpful, because you knew how much you had to do and when you could stop. I liked having the option of the exercises for really busy days, because you don't have to get changed for them. I also liked the walking, because my husband could come too, but I found the isocises the hardest because I kept forgetting to keep breathing while holding the tension!'

### Liz, 43, housewife:

'I would probably have scored all my points from walking and exercises if I hadn't been able to persuade a neighbour to start jogging with me. But we took the first tentative steps together, and it wasn't anywhere near as difficult as I expected. We walked for five minutes first, then broke into a jog for one minute, then walked for another five. Afterwards, we had to work out how many points we got for the walking and how many for jogging. Then, over the first three weeks, we were able to jog for longer, so our points score went up accordingly.

'Having to increase the amount of exercise you do to keep pace with the graduated scores needed each week seemed a good idea because it provided the right sort of incentive. Sometimes I felt a bit stiff if I'd jogged a lot the day before, but if I jogged again, it seemed to disappear. Also, I only realised in the third week that I could have counted my walks to and from the shops, and with the dog, as part of my points-scoring exercise too, so I did more than was necessary at first.'

### Karen, 33, office manager:

'I had tried jogging on and off for years, but there was never any real incentive before to keep at it. I didn't want to run in marathons or fun runs, I just wanted to keep fit, but when winter came it usually seemed less inviting to go out jogging. I kept telling myself I'd go out the next day. Using the tables changed all that, because then I kept thinking that if I didn't go out to jog on Tuesday, and I was going out socially on Wednesday evening, then I'd never reach my points score that week. So I'd get out on Tuesday even if I didn't feel like it, whereas before I probably wouldn't have bothered. The strange thing is that once you're out you feel so much better and wonder why you were so reluctant in the first place, and then you're really pleased that you decided to make the effort.'

### Sophie, 18, student:

'Everyone I knew seemed to be on some form of star-vation diet, forever miserable because they couldn't eat anything and constantly hungry. So they were all surprised whenever I'd suddenly announce that I'd just got to walk round the block to complete my weekly points total. None of them seemed to have considered a structured exercise programme as a way of achieving the type of results they wanted. In fact, they'd all said "Oh, exercise, boring!" when I first started.

'But, probably because they saw me becoming so involved in what I was doing, constantly adding up my projected points scores, and yet so happy to be doing something which in itself provides a great deal of satisfaction – which, let's face it, a starvation diet doesn't – they soon all wanted copies of the tables.'

# $-7-$

By now I hope that you will be straining at the leash to get started! So let me explain how the tables work, and how to use them.

For each of the activities outlined in Chapter 5 I have devised a simple points-scoring system, which rewards the amount and regularity of your exercising. The further you jog or walk, and the more often you perform the exercises or isocises, the more points you earn.

The target I am setting you is to reach a specific points total for each of the 10 weeks in the programme. You can achieve that total by choosing any combination of the various points-scoring activities you wish. For example, you could jog on a Monday, walk on a Tuesday, and do exercises and isocises on a Wednesday. Or you could do all four on one day. Every part of the exercise programme is rewarded with its own designated points score, and you simply add them together to try to reach your total. To help you keep track, separate check charts for each of the 10 weeks appear on pages 107–117, and you can fill these in day by day.

For Week 1, your target total is 100 points. That works out at an average of less than 15 points per day, which should be well within your reach. For example, you could earn those daily 15 points by simply walking for a quarter of an hour. Or by performing just one set of the exercises outlined on page 56. Then each week the target is raised by 100 points. For the second week it is 200 points, in the third week it is 300 points, and so on.

On the horizon, at the end of Week 10, is the Grand Slam, which is to achieve a total of 1,000 points!

That target may seem impossibly out of reach to you at present. But if you can hit those gradually climbing intermediate targets week by week it will soon become perfectly attainable. Remember, I am not trying to put in front of you a challenge which is impossible; what would be the point? On the other hand, it needs to be at a level which will still give you considerable personal satisfaction in meeting it. Not only that, but will you still recognise yourself in the mirror?

## THE TABLES

The points tables are set out on pages 79–105, and you will notice that there are five separate columns. The first column contains the number of points you are awarded, from 1 to 150, in return for the amount you complete of each of the four physical activities. You will come to know these tables pretty well after just a week or so!

### Jogging

The second column relates to Jogging, and shows the total time you need to spend jogging in order to earn the points score on that line. For example, if you jogged for 2 minutes, you would receive 4 points; if you jogged for 8 minutes, you would receive 16 points, and so on. The tables go up to a score of 150 points, which is awarded to jogging for 75 minutes. At the end of each day you can then enter your total jogging points into your weekly check chart (pages 107–117).

Clearly, in the early days you should only be looking at the lower points scores. But as weeks pass and you become fitter, you will find yourself progressing up the table to higher scores with increasingly longer continuous jogs for no greater effort. Remember, you are not trying to break records by jogging faster; you are simply trying to maintain the same, comfortable 'conversation' pace, but going further. And as your legs gain stamina, it really will become easier rather than harder.

But in that opening week or two, you may well decide to adopt the jog-walk-jog method of getting fit for jogging, where you jog for 20 seconds and walk for 30, as explained on page 52. If you do, it is perfectly acceptable to score your points for the overall time you spend jogging and walking as if it were all jogging. In due course, it *will* be all jogging, because as you become fitter you will notice that not only is there no longer any need to slow to a walk any more, but to do so would actually interrupt your rhythm.

## Walking

This is the simplest table of all to follow, because each minute of walking gains one point, e.g. 18 points for 18 minutes' walking, up to 150 points for 2½ hours (150 minutes) of walking. You can include any walking during the day (such as walking to the shops, or to post a letter) in your points-scoring total, although easily the most effective walking for your fitness will be a continuous, brisk pace.

The advantage of including walking in the points-scoring programme is that some days you may really not feel like jogging, but you could manage a walk instead. So just getting you out of the house and taking exercise, even if it doesn't raise your pulse as high as jogging or have as direct an effect on your gluteal muscles, is still worth a reasonable points score.

## Exercises

Points for the exercise programme are awarded for the number of times you complete a full set of the exercises, or part of the set, laid out on pages 56–58.

There are six different exercises, and they all have to be performed with the correct number of repetitions to constitute the 'one full set' which would earn you 15 points on the tables. If you perform two full sets, the score rises to 30 points. For three full sets, it is 45 points, and so on. But the tables also allow you to perform just part of the full set, too. For example, doing any two of the exercises (with the correct number of repetitions) still earns you five points. Most other possible combinations are included in the tables (e.g. four full sets, plus three individual exercises performed for a fifth time, brings you 67 points).

*Isocises*

A similar points-scoring system applies to the isocises. However, as there are only four separate isocises, you need to perform a greater number of full sets than the exercises to earn the same points. For example, four full sets of exercises will earn 60 points, but you need six full sets of isocises for the same number of points.

## GENERAL

• The tables allocate points scores for up to 10 full sets of exercises, and 15 full sets of isocises (and can be extended to an indefinite number). However, while I do not anticipate that you would want to perform as many sets of exercises or isocises in one single session, these activities do lend themselves to further repetition at various times of the day. So score the total number of sets you have achieved by the end of the day.

• Equating fairly the points-scoring for the jogging/walking with the exercises/isocises was tricky, and in the end partly based upon the total estimated time taken to perform the exercises/isocises. This was to avoid any accusations that it was much quicker to earn points with these indoor activities.

• The richest source of points-scoring is the jogging section, because that is the exercise which will do you most good in terms of trimming and slimming. Jogging also needs a conscious planning decision, and usually involves getting changed before and after, aspects which deserve to be reflected in the points scoring.

It also greatly improves your cardiovascular fitness (as to a lesser extent does walking), an aspect to which the exercises and isocises scarcely contribute. They are, however, very good for toning up specific muscles, and have the advantage that they can be performed at short notice practically anywhere. If you need to score points quickly, as when you suddenly find you have less time available than you thought, the exercises/isocises are the handy solution.

• There is no doubt, though, that the most effective way of achieving your goal is through a sensible combination of all four activities. Scoring all your points through, say, exercises alone is theoretically possible, but to do so would have a much less beneficial effect on your shape and fitness than incorporating a solid proportion of jogging and walking.

## POINTS PLANNING

What is the best way to plan your points scoring? After all, you will not want to reach Friday evening and only then discover that you still have to earn a vast number of points to fulfil your weekly target. Using the weekly check chart (pages 107–117) can be extremely helpful not only as a way of recording what you have actually achieved, but also as an advance planner, like a diary. Once you have decided when you wish to start your 10-week programme, you can fill in the dates of each week at the head of the relevant page in the check chart.

Beneath the weekly target total on each page, I have indicated the approximate daily average points score you will need to maintain to reach the target. However, that is based on a seven-day week and some people may find that they have to achieve their score within fewer days. Certainly, most runners have one rest day a week on which they do not train, as a period of mental and physical recovery. So if there are days when you have appointments or other commitments which might reduce your points-scoring opportunities, write them in pencil on the chart as a reminder, and treat them as possible rest days.

Then you can plan exactly how you intend to earn the necessary points. To reach the points target of 300 in Week 3, for example, you need an average daily total of 43 points. Looking at the tables, you could earn those 43 points by jogging for 21½ minutes, or by walking for 43 minutes, or by performing three full sets of the exercises, or by four full sets (plus one) of the isocises. Alternatively, you could earn 43 points by a combination of those activities, such as jogging for 10 minutes (20 points) and doing two full sets of the exercises (plus one) for the remaining 23 points. The different combinations are endless – but a little planning is important.

Some people do prefer exercising first, such as jogging until they are tired, and only then looking at their watch. Then they check the tables to see how many points they have scored. By midweek, of course, they still have to work out how many points they now require for their target, and only then do they plan the exact details of their remaining exercise sessions.

## REMEMBER TO REST!

The image of an Olympic athlete is often that of someone with boundless energy, who is superbly fit and constantly on the go. However, in reality, the Olympic athlete is someone who is usually tired and aching from their constantly high level of training. While the level of physical activity within this programme is relatively modest by comparison, it will still be a new experience to many of those undertaking the 1,000-point challenge.

In order to maintain progress, and meet the gently increasing demands of the exercise, getting proper rest is essential. The process of achieving a new level of fitness can be very rewarding, but also somewhat tiring. However, maintaining it once you are fit is much less demanding. Thus, give yourself the best possible chance of succeeding in reaching the 1,000-point challenge by allowing your body to recover properly from its work. That may mean going to bed an hour earlier than usual, or cutting down temporarily on other commitments where possible.

## WHAT NEXT?
Does it all end after you have achieved 1,000 points in a week? Not at all. Having worked so hard in order to attain your new level of fitness, it would be an enormous shame if it all just faded away. So when you achieve the 1,000 points total, take a few days to congratulate yourself, and then consider new targets. And, particularly, higher scores. The chance to achieve a personal best performance is the driving force for most sportsmen, and to maintain your own high standard you could pick a week in which you try to improve your own personal best exercise score.

There is no need to worry that the tables in this book finish at 150 points for each activity. At the foot of the tables there is a key which will enable you to extend each column to infinity should you wish.

But now it's up to you. I have told you the whys and the wherefores of getting yourself back into shape, and given you the blueprint for a New You. I can't, however, get out there and do it for you.

One of the most satisfying aspects of being involved with a project like this is knowing that it can work for you and everybody else if only you will allow it to. If you can commit yourself to the initial 10-week period, aiming for each weekly target in turn and eating sensibly, I would like to think that at the end of those 10 short weeks you will have only one question to ask: 'Why on earth didn't someone tell me about this years ago?'

Now that they have, how about scoring your first points right now?

# THE TEMPLE TABLES

| POINTS SCORE | JOGGING | WALKING | EXERCISES | ISOCISES |
|---|---|---|---|---|
| 1 | 30 secs | 1 min | | |
| 2 | 1 min | 2 mins | | |
| 3 | 1.5 mins | 3 mins | any 1 exercise | any 1 isocise |
| 4 | 2 mins | 4 mins | | |
| 5 | 2.5 mins | 5 mins | any 2 exercises | any 2 isocises |
| 6 | 3 mins | 6 mins | | |

| POINTS SCORE | JOGGING | WALKING | EXERCISES | ISOCISES |
| --- | --- | --- | --- | --- |
| 7 | 3.5 mins | 7 mins | any 3 exercises | any 3 isocises |
| 8 | 4 mins | 8 mins | | |
| 9 | 4.5 mins | 9 mins | any 4 exercises | |
| 10 | 5 mins | 10 mins | | 1 full set of isocises |
| 11 | 5.5 mins | 11 mins | | |
| 12 | 6 mins | 12 mins | any 5 exercises | |

| POINTS SCORE | JOGGING | WALKING | EXERCISES | ISOCISES |
|---|---|---|---|---|
| 13 | 6.5 mins | 13 mins | | 1 full set of isocises, plus 1 |
| 14 | 7 mins | 14 mins | | |
| 15 | 7.5 mins | 15 mins | 1 full set of exercises | 1 full set of isocises, plus 2 |
| 16 | 8 mins | 16 mins | | |
| 17 | 8.5 mins | 17 mins | | 1 full set of isocises, plus 3 |
| 18 | 9 mins | 18 mins | 1 full set of exercises, plus 1 | |

| POINTS SCORE | JOGGING | WALKING | EXERCISES | ISOCISES |
|---|---|---|---|---|
| **19** | 9.5 mins | 19 mins | | |
| **20** | 10 mins | 20 mins | 1 full set of exercises, plus 2 | 2 full sets of of isocises |
| **21** | 10.5 mins | 21 mins | | |
| **22** | 11 mins | 22 mins | 1 full set of exercises, plus 3 | |
| **23** | 11.5 mins | 23 mins | | 2 full sets of isocises, plus 1 |
| **24** | 12 mins | 24 mins | 1 full set of exercises, plus 4 | |

| POINTS SCORE | JOGGING | WALKING | EXERCISES | ISOCISES |
| --- | --- | --- | --- | --- |
| **25** | 12.5 mins | 25 mins | | 2 full sets of isocises, plus 2 |
| **26** | 13 mins | 26 mins | | |
| **27** | 13.5 mins | 27 mins | 1 full set of exercises, plus 5 | 2 full sets of isocises, plus 3 |
| **28** | 14 mins | 28 mins | | |
| **29** | 14.5 mins | 29 mins | | |
| **30** | 15 mins | 30 mins | 2 full sets of exercises | 3 full sets of isocises |

| POINTS SCORE | JOGGING | WALKING | EXERCISES | ISOCISES |
|---|---|---|---|---|
| **31** | 15.5 mins | 31 mins | | |
| **32** | 16 mins | 32 mins | | |
| **33** | 16.5 mins | 33 mins | 2 full sets of exercises, plus 1 | 3 full sets of isocises, plus 1 |
| **34** | 17 mins | 34 mins | | |
| **35** | 17.5 mins | 35 mins | 2 full sets of exercises, plus 2 | 3 full sets of isocises, plus 2 |
| **36** | 18 mins | 36 mins | | |

| POINTS SCORE | JOGGING | WALKING | EXERCISES | ISOCISES |
|---|---|---|---|---|
| **37** | 18.5 mins | 37 mins | 2 full sets of exercises, plus 3 | 3 full sets of isocises, plus 3 |
| **38** | 19 mins | 38 mins | | |
| **39** | 19.5 mins | 39 mins | 2 full sets of exercises, plus 4 | |
| **40** | 20 mins | 40 mins | | 4 full sets of isocises |
| **41** | 20.5 mins | 41 mins | | |
| **42** | 21 mins | 42 mins | 2 full sets of exercises, plus 5 | |

| POINTS SCORE | JOGGING | WALKING | EXERCISES | ISOCISES |
| --- | --- | --- | --- | --- |
| **43** | 21.5 mins | 43 mins | | 4 full sets of isocises, plus 1 |
| **44** | 22 mins | 44 mins | | |
| **45** | 22.5 mins | 45 mins | 3 full sets of exercises | 4 full sets of isocises, plus 2 |
| **46** | 23 mins | 46 mins | | |
| **47** | 23.5 mins | 47 mins | | 4 full sets of isocises, plus 3 |
| **48** | 24 mins | 48 mins | 3 full sets of exercises, plus 1 | |

| POINTS SCORE | JOGGING | WALKING | EXERCISES | ISOCISES |
|---|---|---|---|---|
| **49** | 24.5 mins | 49 mins | | |
| **50** | 25 mins | 50 mins | 3 full sets of exercises, plus 2 | 5 full sets of isocises |
| **51** | 25.5 mins | 51 mins | | |
| **52** | 26 mins | 52 mins | 3 full sets of exercises, plus 3 | |
| **53** | 26.5 mins | 53 mins | | 5 full sets of isocises, plus 1 |
| **54** | 27 mins | 54 mins | 3 full sets of exercises, plus 4 | |

| POINTS SCORE | JOGGING | WALKING | EXERCISES | ISOCISES |
|---|---|---|---|---|
| **55** | 27.5 mins | 55 mins | | 5 full sets of isocises, plus 2 |
| **56** | 28 mins | 56 mins | | |
| **57** | 28.5 mins | 57 mins | 3 full sets of exercises, plus 5 | 5 full sets of isocises, plus 3 |
| **58** | 29 mins | 58 mins | | |
| **59** | 29.5 mins | 59 mins | | |
| **60** | 30 mins | 60 mins | 4 full sets of exercises | 6 full sets of isocises |

| POINTS SCORE | JOGGING | WALKING | EXERCISES | ISOCISES |
|---|---|---|---|---|
| **61** | 30.5 mins | 61 mins | | |
| **62** | 31 mins | 62 mins | | |
| **63** | 31.5 mins | 63 mins | 4 full sets of exercises, plus 1 | 6 full sets of isocises, plus 1 |
| **64** | 32 mins | 64 mins | | |
| **65** | 32.5 mins | 65 mins | 4 full sets of exercises, plus 2 | 6 full sets of isocises, plus 2 |
| **66** | 33 mins | 66 mins | | |

| POINTS SCORE | JOGGING | WALKING | EXERCISES | ISOCISES |
|---|---|---|---|---|
| **67** | 33.5 mins | 67 mins | 4 full sets of exercises, plus 3 | 6 full sets of isocises, plus 3 |
| **68** | 34 mins | 68 mins | | |
| **69** | 34.5 mins | 69 mins | 4 full sets of exercises, plus 4 | |
| **70** | 35 mins | 70 mins | | 7 full sets of isocises |
| **71** | 35.5 mins | 71 mins | | |
| **72** | 36 mins | 72 mins | 4 full sets of exercises, plus 5 | |

| POINTS SCORE | JOGGING | WALKING | EXERCISES | ISOCISES |
| --- | --- | --- | --- | --- |
| **73** | 36.5 mins | 73 mins | | 7 full sets of isocises, plus 1 |
| **74** | 37 mins | 74 mins | | |
| **75** | 37.5 mins | 75 mins | 5 full sets of exercises | 7 full sets of isocises, plus 2 |
| **76** | 38 mins | 76 mins | | |
| **77** | 38.5 mins | 77 mins | | 7 full sets of isocises, plus 3 |
| **78** | 39 mins | 78 mins | | |

| POINTS SCORE | JOGGING | WALKING | EXERCISES | ISOCISES |
|---|---|---|---|---|
| 79 | 39.5 mins | 79 mins | | |
| 80 | 40 mins | 80 mins | 5 full sets of exercises, plus 2 | 8 full sets of isocises |
| 81 | 40.5 mins | 81 mins | | |
| 82 | 41 mins | 82 mins | 5 full sets of exercises, plus 3 | |
| 83 | 41.5 mins | 83 mins | | 8 full sets of isocises, plus 1 |
| 84 | 42 mins | 84 mins | | |

| POINTS SCORE | JOGGING | WALKING | EXERCISES | ISOCISES |
|---|---|---|---|---|
| **85** | 42.5 mins | 85 mins | | 8 full sets of isocises, plus 2 |
| **86** | 43 mins | 86 mins | | |
| **87** | 43.5 mins | 87 mins | 5 full sets of exercises, plus 5 | 8 full sets of isocises, plus 3 |
| **88** | 44 mins | 88 mins | | |
| **89** | 44.5 mins | 89 mins | | |
| **90** | 45 mins | 90 mins | 6 full sets of exercises | 9 full sets of isocises |

| POINTS SCORE | JOGGING | WALKING | EXERCISES | ISOCISES |
|---|---|---|---|---|
| **91** | 45.5 mins | 91 mins | | |
| **92** | 46 mins | 92 mins | | |
| **93** | 46.5 mins | 93 mins | 6 full sets of exercises, plus 1 | 9 full sets of isocises, plus 1 |
| **94** | 47 mins | 94 mins | | |
| **95** | 47.5 mins | 95 mins | 6 full sets of exercises, plus 2 | 9 full sets of isocises, plus 2 |
| **96** | 48 mins | 96 mins | | |

| POINTS SCORE | JOGGING | WALKING | EXERCISES | ISOCISES |
|---|---|---|---|---|
| **97** | 48.5 mins | 97 mins | 6 full sets of exercises, plus 3 | 9 full sets of isocises, plus 3 |
| **98** | 49 mins | 98 mins | | |
| **99** | 49.5 mins | 99 mins | 6 full sets of exercises, plus 4 | |
| **100** | 50 mins | 100 mins | | 10 full sets of isocises |
| **101** | 50.5 mins | 101 mins | | |
| **102** | 51 mins | 102 mins | 6 full sets of exercises, plus 5 | |

| POINTS SCORE | JOGGING | WALKING | EXERCISES | ISOCISES |
|---|---|---|---|---|
| **103** | 51.5 mins | 103 mins | | 10 full sets of isocises, plus 1 |
| **104** | 52 mins | 104 mins | | |
| **105** | 52.5 mins | 105 mins | 7 full sets of exercises | 10 full sets of isocises, plus 2 |
| **106** | 53 mins | 106 mins | | |
| **107** | 53.5 mins | 107 mins | | 10 full sets of isocises, plus 3 |
| **108** | 54 mins | 108 mins | 7 full sets of exercises, plus 1 | |

| POINTS SCORE | JOGGING | WALKING | EXERCISES | ISOCISES |
| --- | --- | --- | --- | --- |
| **109** | 54.5 mins | 109 mins | | |
| **110** | 55 mins | 110 mins | 7 full sets of exercises, plus 2 | 11 full sets of isocises |
| **111** | 55.5 mins | 111 mins | | |
| **112** | 56 mins | 112 mins | 7 full sets of exercises, plus 3 | |
| **113** | 56.5 mins | 113 mins | | 11 full sets of isocises, plus 1 |
| **114** | 57 mins | 114 mins | 7 full sets of exercises, plus 4 | |

| POINTS SCORE | JOGGING | WALKING | EXERCISES | ISOCISES |
|---|---|---|---|---|
| **115** | 57.5 mins | 115 mins | | 11 full sets of isocises, plus 2 |
| **116** | 58 mins | 116 mins | | |
| **117** | 58.5 mins | 117 mins | 7 full sets of exercises, plus 5 | 11 full sets of isocises, plus 3 |
| **118** | 59 mins | 118 mins | | |
| **119** | 59.5 mins | 119 mins | | |
| **120** | 60 mins | 120 mins | 8 full sets of exercises | 12 full sets of isocises |

| POINTS SCORE | JOGGING | WALKING | EXERCISES | ISOCISES |
|---|---|---|---|---|
| **121** | 60.5 mins | 121 mins | | |
| **122** | 61 mins | 122 mins | | |
| **123** | 61.5 mins | 123 mins | 8 full sets of exercises, plus 1 | 12 full sets of isocises, plus 1 |
| **124** | 62 mins | 124 mins | | |
| **125** | 62.5 mins | 125 mins | 8 full sets of exercises, plus 2 | 12 full sets of isocises, plus 2 |
| **126** | 63 mins | 126 mins | | |

| POINTS SCORE | JOGGING | WALKING | EXERCISES | ISOCISES |
| --- | --- | --- | --- | --- |
| **127** | 63.5 mins | 127 mins | 8 full sets of exercises, plus 3 | 12 full sets of isocises, plus 3 |
| **128** | 64 mins | 128 mins | | |
| **129** | 64.5 mins | 129 mins | 8 full sets of exercises, plus 4 | |
| **130** | 65 mins | 130 mins | | 13 full sets of isocises |
| **131** | 65.5 mins | 131 mins | | |
| **132** | 66 mins | 132 mins | 8 full sets of exercises, plus 5 | |

| POINTS SCORE | JOGGING | WALKING | EXERCISES | ISOCISES |
|---|---|---|---|---|
| **133** | 66.5 mins | 133 mins | | 13 full sets of isocises, plus 1 |
| **134** | 67 mins | 134 mins | | |
| **135** | 67.5 mins | 135 mins | 9 full sets of exercises | 13 full sets of isocises, plus 2 |
| **136** | 68 mins | 136 mins | | |
| **137** | 68.5 mins | 137 mins | | 13 full sets of isocises, plus 3 |
| **138** | 69 mins | 138 mins | 9 full sets of exercises, plus 1 | |

| POINTS SCORE | JOGGING | WALKING | EXERCISES | ISOCISES |
|---|---|---|---|---|
| **139** | 69.5 mins | 139 mins | | |
| **140** | 70 mins | 140 mins | 9 full sets of exercises, plus 2 | 14 full sets of isocises |
| **141** | 70.5 mins | 141 mins | | |
| **142** | 71 mins | 142 mins | 9 full sets of exercises, plus 3 | |
| **143** | 71.5 mins | 143 mins | | 14 full sets of isocises, plus 1 |
| **144** | 72 mins | 144 mins | 9 full sets of exercises, plus 4 | |

| POINTS SCORE | JOGGING | WALKING | EXERCISES | ISOCISES |
|---|---|---|---|---|
| **145** | 72.5 mins | 145 mins | | 14 full sets of isocises, plus 2 |
| **146** | 73 mins | 146 mins | | |
| **147** | 73.5 mins | 147 mins | 9 full sets of exercises, plus 5 | 14 full sets of isocises, plus 3 |
| **148** | 74 mins | 148 mins | | |
| **149** | 74.5 mins | 149 mins | | |
| **150** | 75 mins | 150 mins | 10 full sets of exercises | 15 full sets of isocises |

| POINTS SCORE | JOGGING | WALKING | EXERCISES | ISOCISES |
| --- | --- | --- | --- | --- |
| **To continue:** | add 2 points per minute of jogging | add 1 point per minute of walking | add 15 points per full set of exercises | add 10 points per full set of isocises |
| | | | | |
| | | | | |
| | | | | |
| | | | | |

# WEEKLY CHECK CHARTS

# WEEK 1

**Dates: From** _____ **to** _____

TARGET: 100 POINTS (average 14.3 per day)

POINTS SCORED

| DAY | JOGGING | WALKING | EXERCISES | ISOCISES | DAILY AGGREGATE |
|-----|---------|---------|-----------|----------|-----------------|
| **SUNDAY** | | | | | |
| **MONDAY** | | | | | |
| **TUESDAY** | | | | | |
| **WEDNESDAY** | | | | | |
| **THURSDAY** | | | | | |
| **FRIDAY** | | | | | |
| **SATURDAY** | | | | | |
| | | | | **WEEKLY TOTAL ACHIEVED** | |

# WEEK 2

**Dates: From** _____ **to** _____

TARGET: 200 POINTS (average 28.6 per day)

POINTS SCORED

| DAY | JOGGING | WALKING | EXERCISES | ISOCISES | DAILY AGGREGATE |
|-----|---------|---------|-----------|----------|-----------------|
| **SUNDAY** | | | | | |
| **MONDAY** | | | | | |
| **TUESDAY** | | | | | |
| **WEDNESDAY** | | | | | |
| **THURSDAY** | | | | | |
| **FRIDAY** | | | | | |
| **SATURDAY** | | | | | |
| | | | | **WEEKLY TOTAL ACHIEVED** | |

# WEEK 3

**Dates: From** _____ **to** _____

TARGET: 300 POINTS (average 42.9 per day)

POINTS SCORED

| DAY | JOGGING | WALKING | EXERCISES | ISOCISES | DAILY AGGREGATE |
|-----|---------|---------|-----------|----------|-----------------|
| **SUNDAY** | | | | | |
| **MONDAY** | | | | | |
| **TUESDAY** | | | | | |
| **WEDNESDAY** | | | | | |
| **THURSDAY** | | | | | |
| **FRIDAY** | | | | | |
| **SATURDAY** | | | | | |
| | | | | **WEEKLY TOTAL ACHIEVED** | |

# WEEK 4

**Dates: From _____ to _____**

TARGET: 400 POINTS (average 57.2 per day)

POINTS SCORED

| DAY | JOGGING | WALKING | EXERCISES | ISOCISES | DAILY AGGREGATE |
|---|---|---|---|---|---|
| **SUNDAY** | | | | | |
| **MONDAY** | | | | | |
| **TUESDAY** | | | | | |
| **WEDNESDAY** | | | | | |
| **THURSDAY** | | | | | |
| **FRIDAY** | | | | | |
| **SATURDAY** | | | | | |
| | | | | **WEEKLY TOTAL ACHIEVED** | |

# WEEK 5

**Dates: From** _____ **to** _____

TARGET: 500 POINTS (average 71.4 per day)

POINTS SCORED

| DAY | JOGGING | WALKING | EXERCISES | ISOCISES | DAILY AGGREGATE |
|---|---|---|---|---|---|
| **SUNDAY** | | | | | |
| **MONDAY** | | | | | |
| **TUESDAY** | | | | | |
| **WEDNESDAY** | | | | | |
| **THURSDAY** | | | | | |
| **FRIDAY** | | | | | |
| **SATURDAY** | | | | | |
| | | | | **WEEKLY TOTAL ACHIEVED** | |

# WEEK 6

**Dates: From** _____ **to** _____

TARGET: 600 POINTS (average 85.7 per day)

POINTS SCORED

| DAY | JOGGING | WALKING | EXERCISES | ISOCISES | DAILY AGGREGATE |
|-----|---------|---------|-----------|----------|-----------------|
| **SUNDAY** | | | | | |
| **MONDAY** | | | | | |
| **TUESDAY** | | | | | |
| **WEDNESDAY** | | | | | |
| **THURSDAY** | | | | | |
| **FRIDAY** | | | | | |
| **SATURDAY** | | | | | |
| | | | | **WEEKLY TOTAL ACHIEVED** | |

# WEEK 7

**Dates: From** _____ **to** _____

TARGET: 700 POINTS (average 100 per day)

POINTS SCORED

| DAY | JOGGING | WALKING | EXERCISES | ISOCISES | DAILY AGGREGATE |
|---|---|---|---|---|---|
| **SUNDAY** | | | | | |
| **MONDAY** | | | | | |
| **TUESDAY** | | | | | |
| **WEDNESDAY** | | | | | |
| **THURSDAY** | | | | | |
| **FRIDAY** | | | | | |
| **SATURDAY** | | | | | |
| | | | | **WEEKLY TOTAL ACHIEVED** | |

# WEEK 8

**Dates: From** _____ **to** _____

TARGET: 800 POINTS (average 114.3 per day)

POINTS SCORED

| DAY | JOGGING | WALKING | EXERCISES | ISOCISES | DAILY AGGREGATE |
|---|---|---|---|---|---|
| **SUNDAY** | | | | | |
| **MONDAY** | | | | | |
| **TUESDAY** | | | | | |
| **WEDNESDAY** | | | | | |
| **THURSDAY** | | | | | |
| **FRIDAY** | | | | | |
| **SATURDAY** | | | | | |
| | | | | WEEKLY TOTAL ACHIEVED | |

# WEEK 9

**Dates: From** _____ **to** _____

TARGET: 900 POINTS (average 128.6 per day)

POINTS SCORED

| DAY | JOGGING | WALKING | EXERCISES | ISOCISES | DAILY AGGREGATE |
|-----|---------|---------|-----------|----------|-----------------|
| **SUNDAY** | | | | | |
| **MONDAY** | | | | | |
| **TUESDAY** | | | | | |
| **WEDNESDAY** | | | | | |
| **THURSDAY** | | | | | |
| **FRIDAY** | | | | | |
| **SATURDAY** | | | | | |
| | | | | WEEKLY TOTAL ACHIEVED | |

# WEEK 10

**Dates: From** _____ **to** _____

TARGET: 1,000 POINTS (average 142.9 per day)

POINTS SCORED

| DAY | JOGGING | WALKING | EXERCISES | ISOCISES | DAILY AGGREGATE |
|---|---|---|---|---|---|
| **SUNDAY** | | | | | |
| **MONDAY** | | | | | |
| **TUESDAY** | | | | | |
| **WEDNESDAY** | | | | | |
| **THURSDAY** | | | | | |
| **FRIDAY** | | | | | |
| **SATURDAY** | | | | | |
| | | | | WEEKLY TOTAL ACHIEVED | |

# REEBOK
# SPECIALIST CLUBS

## REEBOK
## INSTRUCTOR PROGRAMME

The Reebok Instructor Programme is an active forum for exchanging valuable ideas with fellow teaching professionals at every level nationwide.

Enrolment is free and open to all PROFESSIONAL exercise and fitness instructors. Once enrolled, instructors receive an information package and the right to order shoes direct from Reebok at Special instructor prices.

They will also receive regular copies of the Reebok Instructor News. Contributions from Instructors, Sports Physiologists, Club Managers and other professionals from the fitness world are welcomed. The Reebok Instructor News also contains details of forthcoming seminars, workshops, conferences, exhibitions etc. in the UK, all of particular interest to fitness professionals.

## REEBOK
## RUNNING SISTERS NETWORK

The Reebok Running Sisters network aims to put women runners in touch with other women in their area to run together for fitness, fun and friendship. All ages and standards are welcome, from a total beginner to seasoned marathoner.

The Network is administered by a team of Regional Organisers, all volunteers. Your enquiry will be forwarded to your nearest Regional Organiser who will shortly get in touch with you and where possible match you up with a local runner or group.

No woman is too old, too fat, or too slow to run with the Network. The key to success is starting slowly and building up gently, setting realistic goals and achieving them. You don't have to race to enjoy your running, but it is an ideal way of monitoring your improvement and of meeting and making new friends.

## REEBOK RACING CLUB

The Reebok Racing Club is a worldwide organisation numbering amongst its members such British luminaries as Steve and Hugh Jones and Tim Hutchings. The red, white and navy vest has breasted the tape in the world's foremost road and track events as well as being much in evidence throughout the field in many road races.

The UK Racing Club has been active since 1982 and caters for runners of all standards. Members may enjoy the opportunity of participating in training weekends in some of Britain's most picturesque regions. These weekends are led by world-class athletes. There are also opportunities for club travel to prestigious races in Europe and America in the company of fellow members. Membership also entitles you to a club newsletter with coaching tips from top class athletes and other club news – as well as the opportunity to wear an exclusive line of performance clothing.

**To receive an application form for any of the above clubs, simply call Christian Vity, Marketing Dept., Reebok UK, Tel: 0524 36313.**

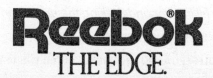

# FOR YOUR RECORD

## Your personal statistics before and after the 10-week programme

|  | BEFORE | AFTER |
|---|---|---|
| Dates of measurement |  |  |
| Weight (pre-breakfast) |  |  |
| Hips |  |  |
| Waist |  |  |
| Thighs |  |  |

*For you to fill in before undertaking the programme:*

PERSONAL TARGET

HOW DID YOU FEEL ABOUT YOURSELF BEFORE YOU STARTED THE 10-WEEK PROGRAMME?

*For you to fill in after undertaking the programme:*

DID YOU ACHIEVE YOUR PERSONAL TARGET?

HOW DID YOU FEEL ABOUT YOURSELF AFTER THE 10-WEEK PROGRAMME?